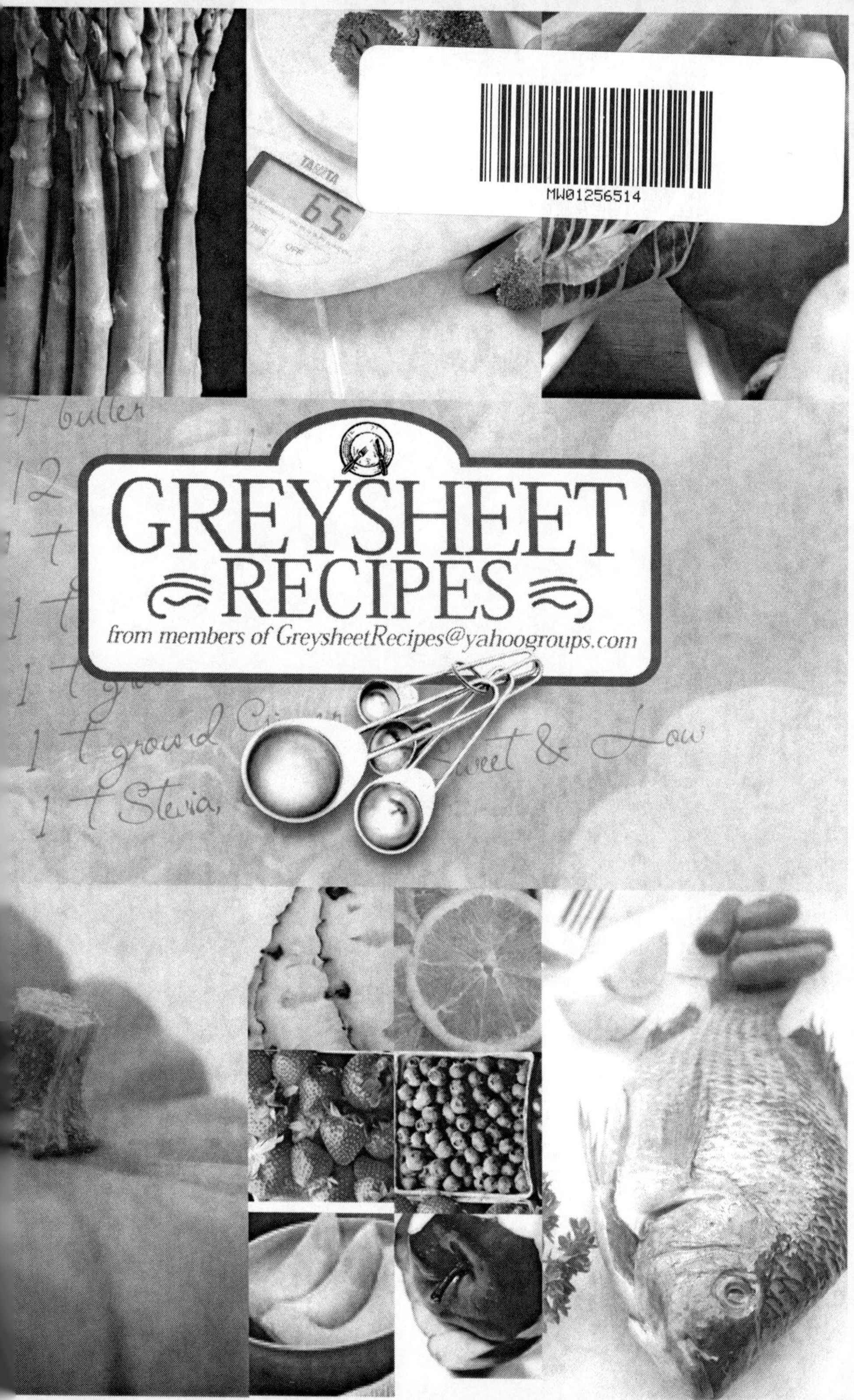
MW01256514
GREYSHEET
RECIPES
from members of GreysheetRecipes@yahoogroups.com

Greysheet Recipes Collection
Edited by Anonymous Member

http://www.greysheetrecipes.org
ISBN 978-0-9725378-4-8

Note: Proceeds from the sale of this book will be donated to
GreySheeters Anonymous World Service Inc.
http://www.greysheet.org

This book is not official literature of
GreySheeters Anonymous (GSA).

Table of Contents

Introduction

Welcome

GreysheetRecipes is an online forum, hosted at YahooGroups.com, founded in 2000 by members of GreySheeters Anonymous. The discussion group is for members to post and discuss recipes that meet the requirements of the food on the Greysheet Food Plan. The purpose of the discussion group is to help members achieve and maintain Greysheet Abstinence. Specific foods may be mentioned. To subscribe to the GreysheetRecipes online forum, send an email to *greysheetrecipes-subscribe@yahoogroups.com*

Recipes in the Greysheet Recipes Collection have been contributed by members of GreysheetRecipes. The Collection was compiled by members of Greysheet Recipes and reviewed by three (3) independent Greysheet members to make sure the recipes conform to the Greysheet Food Plan.

The recipes are for informational common sharing purposes only. It is recommended that members continue to discuss and determine what is abstinent in a recipe and a planned meal according to the Greysheet Food Plan with their individual sponsors. You may download a Free copy of the Greysheet Recipes Collection, or order printed copies for yourself or your group, at *http://www.greysheetrecipes.org*.

The appearance of a recipe in the Greysheet Recipes Collection makes no claim that any other Greysheet member, list moderator or editor, agrees with, disagrees with, recommends or sanctions the recipe or resource.

Our primary purpose is to refrain from compulsive overeating and to help other compulsive overeaters refrain from compulsive overeating.

How to Use These Recipes

You will see the Table of Contents and Recipes have been organized into a few basic groups to correspond with the Greysheet:

Beverages
Fat-Oils-Dressing
Fruits, Fruits with Protein
Cooked Vegetable
Wheat Germ Vegetable
Raw Vegetables
Cooked Vegetables with Protein
Protein

The recipes may either include cooking directions for several portions, or cooking directions for a single portion. You know what your Greysheet weighed and measured food portions are, according to the Greysheet.

Since a Greysheet only comes with a sponsor, the Greysheet Recipes Collection will abide by the practice of not giving out the Greysheet here. You may go to GreySheeters Anonymous World Services (GSA) official website: *http://www.greysheet.org/* to find a sponsor. After you find a sponsor and are using the Greysheet Food Plan, come here to see how all these contributed recipes abide by your Greysheet Food Plan.

So often we have been asked in *greysheetrecipes@yahoo.com* - "send me the recipes!," "I need recipes for cooking vegetables!," "where do I find wheat germ recipes?"

Here in this collection you will find answers. Ideas. We hope you enjoy this sharing.

Beverages

Frappe Tea

Blend with blender on crush.

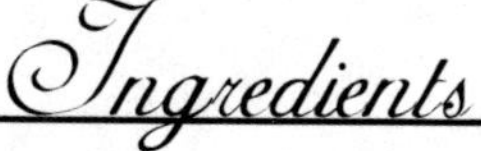

2 tablespoons unsweetened instant tea ◆ 1 cup water ◆ 1 full tray of ice cubes ◆ 2 or more Equal coconut flavoring ◆ lemon juice

Fat-Oil-Dressing

Cole Slaw Salad Dressing

Mix well with shredded cabbage and carrots and toss forever.

Ingredients

1 tsp mayonnaise ◆ 1 oz. mustard ◆ 1/2 tsp sesame oil or peanut oil ◆ 1/2 oz. apple cider vinegar

Dressing, Balsamic Vinegar

Combine all ingredients in a jar. Close lid tightly. Shake vigorously. Measure allotted amount. Keep refrigerated and measure out portion of fat before serving.Measure allotted oil.

Ingredients

3/4 cup olive oil ◆ 1/4 cup balsamic vinegar ◆ 1 shallot, finely chopped ◆ 1/4 teaspoon salt ◆ 1/4 teaspoon freshly ground pepper

Dressing, Cole Slaw

Mix all ingredients together in a jar. Close lid tightly. Shake vigorously. Keep refrigerated and measure out portion of fat before serving.

Ingredients

1 1/2 cup oil ◆ 3 teaspoons onion flakes ◆ 1/2 cup vinegar ◆ 1 teaspoon celery seed ◆ 1 pint real mayonnaise ◆ 3 tablespoons chopped pickle ◆ Several packets of sweetener

Dressing, Tomato

Add your favorite spices to your allowable portion of salad dressing and mix with fork or mixer. Makes 1 serving of fat.

Ingredients

salad dressing ◆ 1/2 ounces tomato paste ◆ 1 teaspoon balsamic vinegar ◆ sweetener to taste ◆ 1/4 cup water

Salad Dressing

Measure allotted amount.

Ingredients

3 teaspoons Mayonnaise ◆ 1/2 oz. Salsa ◆ Add mustard, to taste.

Ketchup

Add all ingredients except equal into a corningware dish (doesn't stain). Measure allotted amount. Cover and microwave on high for 10-15 minutes (depending on the wattage) until thick. Allow to cool to room temperature and add equal sweetener. Keep refrigerated. Measure allotted amount.

Ingredients

1 small can Tomato Paste ◆ 2 small cans Tomato Sauce ◆ 1/4 cup White Vinegar (check with your sponsor) ◆ 1/2 teaspoon Celery Powder ◆ 2 tablespoons dehydrated Onion flakes (check with your sponsor, you can add, extra onion powder if needed) ◆ 2 teaspoon Onion powder ◆ 1 tablespoon Cinnamon Powder ◆ 2 teaspoons Salt ◆ 8 whole Cloves ◆ 1/4 teaspoon Chili Powder ◆ 3/4 cup Water ◆ 6 packets Equal Sweetener

Fruits

Apple Nut Breakfast

Blend cheese, sweetener, and extract with hand mixer, until smooth. Spoon over apple and top with soy nuts before serving.

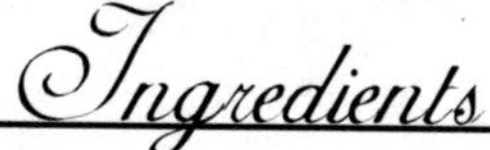

3/8 cup ricotta cheese ◆ 1 ounce roasted ◆ split soy nuts ◆ 1 apple chocolate extract ◆ sweetener

Apple, Baked

Wash and core apples. Arrange in a baking dish in about 1/2 inch water. Spray tops of apples with zero-calorie butter spray. Sprinkle with cinnamon, nutmeg, and sweetener. Bake 30 to 60 minutes at 350 F. The cooking time varies considerably, depending on the texture of the apples. Baste once or twice with the juices in the pan. When done, the apples should be firm and nicely shaped. Serve 1 hot or cold. These taste great heated with sugar-free coffee syrup flavors, such as English Toffee, Raspberry, or Pancake. Measure portion.

Ingredients

peeled and sliced apples ◆ sprinkle of cinnamon ◆ few drops of liquid sweetener ◆ 3/4 cup water

Apples

Combine ingredients and cook in skillet for approximately 10 minutes on medium heat. Cool, bag and freeze. Measure portion.

Ingredients

peeled and sliced apples ◆ sprinkle of cinnamon ◆ few drops of liquid sweetener ◆ 3/4 cup water

Applesauce Cake

Mix all ingredients in a bowl. Bake in a small loaf pan sprayed liberally with Pam or other spray for one hour at 350.

Ingredients

8oz applesauce-no sugar added ◆ 2oz soy flour ◆ 1 egg ◆ sweetener ◆ flavoring to your liking

Apricots

Simply dip apricots in water and eat fresh! Few fruits are better than fresh apricots! They have a rich, smooth flavor and a lovely perfume.

Ingredients

3 medium ripe apricots

Apricots, Poached

Halve the apricots. Crack some of the pits and remove the kernels. Bring water to a boil. Add vanilla, fruit, kernels, and poach till the apricots are just tender. Serve cold.

Ingredients

3 medium apricots ◆ 2 cups water ◆ 1/2 teaspoon vanilla extract

Baked Apple

Remove core from apple. Place apple in dish and sprinkle with cinnamon. Cover apple with soda to middle of apple. Bake at 350 degrees for 1 hour, turning apple over after ½ hour (or microwave for 8 minutes). Apple should be very soft when done. Bake or Microwave

Ingredients

1 large apple ◆ diet raspberry or black cherry soda ◆ cinnamon

Blueberries and Soy

Weigh and measure blueberries. Warm in the microwave until hot and super juicy, then I add 2oz Soy Nut and Soy Butter (I save my other 2oz for another Protein). It's like PBJ

Ingredients

4oz Frozen Blueberries ◆ 2oz Soy Nut and Soy Butter

Blueberry Sauce

Mix ingredients, cook in small pot, bring to boil.

Ingredients

1/2 cup blueberries ◆ 1 packet sweetener ◆ 2 tablespoons cold water

Broiled Orange or Grapefruit

Take orange, cut in half and section like a grapefruit. Add sweetener or flavoring to taste. Broil for 2 minutes under broiler or heat in microwave for 2 minutes

Ingredients

Orange ◆ cut in half ◆ sweetener or flavoring to taste

Cantaloupe with Salt & Lemon

Combine ingredients

Ingredients

8 ozs cantaloupe ◆ 1 tsp fresh squeezed lemon ◆ 1 dash salt from a salt shaker

Cereal with Fruit

Just before serving, mix together.Measure portion.

Ingredients

3/4 cup milk mixed with 1 tablespoon vanilla ◆ 2 oz. granular TVP ◆ 1/2 oz. soy nuts ◆ 1 cup or 8 oz. chopped fruit

Cooking Cranberries

Wash cranberries and pick over for stems and bad ones. Put good cranberries in a Pyrex dish with a lid. Sprinkle them lightly with water and orange zest, a bit of cinnamon, cloves, and nutmeg. Cook them in the microwave 8 to 9 minutes (or on stovetop) until they burst and then mash them up and add some sweetener. Measure & serve.

Ingredients

cranberries ◆ water ◆ orange zest ◆ cinnamon ◆ cloves ◆ nutmeg

Cranberries and Pineapple

Put cranberries in pot on stove and cover with water. Add spices and sweetener. Cook until soft. Add pineapple and mix together. Measure and serve. Store in the refrigerator.

Ingredients

1 bag fresh cranberries ◆ 1 cup crushed pineapple in its own juice ◆ cinnamon or other spices you prefer ◆ sweetener

Frozen Fruits

I like to cut up apples, ripe peaches, plums and apricots and freeze them...takes forever to suck on them for breakfast!

Ingredients

Apples ◆ Peaches ◆ Plums ◆ Apricots

Cranberry, Apple and Pineapple Mix

Put cranberries in a pot, add just enough water to float all the cranberries, and bring to a boil. Meanwhile, cut up 2 or 3 baking apples and put in pot with cranberries. Simmer 5 to 10 minutes. Remove from heat and stir in 1 can drained pineapple chunks. Let the mix cool before refrigerating. Measure & serve.

Ingredients

2 packages fresh cranberries ◆ 2 or 3 baking apples, cut up ◆ 1 cup pineapple

Fruit Salad

Chop apples, peaches, and oranges into 1-inch cubes or pieces. Put all chopped fruit into large bowl. Add can of pineapple. Fold fruit together, to mix. Do not stir too quickly, or pineapple will make it frothy. Refrigerate. Lasts several days in refrigerator. Measure 1 cup to make 1 fruit. If you use blackberries, blueberries, or raspberries, 1 serving of fruit = 1/2 cup, not 1 cup.

Ingredients

2 apples ◆ 3 peaches ◆ 2 oranges, peeled ◆ 1 pint strawberries ◆ 1 cup pineapple ◆ sliced or in chunks, in its own juice

Fruit Staple

Cut up all kinds of apples. Put on ceramic or glass flat dish for 12 minutes or so in the microwave, then put cinnamon on it and bake in the oven at a low temperature. The pieces become small and crisp. Measure portion.

Ingredients

cut up apples ◆ cinnamon

Gooseberry Fool

Pick the stems and tails from the gooseberries. Wash thoroughly and drain. Bring water to a boil in a saucepan. Add berries and simmer until they are just cooked through but not mushy. Stir them and shake the pan from time to time. Let cool. When cool, drain well and put berries through food processor. Stir gooseberry puree into ricotta cheese and sweetener and sugar-free coffee syrup or extract. Chill thoroughly before serving. Measure portion.

Ingredients

1 cup gooseberries ◆ 1/2 cup ricotta cheese ◆ sweetener ◆ sugar-free coffee syrup or extract ◆ 3 cups water

Grapefruit, Broiled

Pull apart sections of grapefruit. Place on a cookie sheet. Spray with zero-calorie butter spray. Top with sweetener. Broil about 5 inches from the heating unit till the fruit is well heated. Serve.

Ingredients

1/2 grapefruit ◆ zero-calorie butter spray sweetener

Great Baked Apple

Cover Apple with Soda to middle of Apple about 1/2 Cup or more soda.

Ingredients

1 Large Apple ◆ core removed, cinnamon to taste
◆ diet Raspberry or Black Cherry Soda

Melon and Ham

Slice ham paper thin. Layer with slices of melon. Top with pepper, and serve.

Ingredients

4 ounces Prosciutto ◆ Smithfield, or Parma Ham ◆ 1/2 cantaloupe or
1/4 casaba or honeydew melon ◆ pepper

Nice Cream

Put all ingredients in a blender, and blend until mixed thoroughly. Turn on your yogurt maker, so the frozen bowl is spinning. Pour the mixture into the top hole of the frozen yogurt maker. Let the yogurt maker spin until the blade no longer moves the mixture. This can be served immediately or stored frozen. A summer favorite! Measure & serve.

Ingredients

1/4 cup cottage cheese or 1/2 cup plain yogurt ◆ 1 cup milk ◆ 1 cup frozen strawberries ◆ peaches, or 1 chilled ◆ peeled apple, or 1/2 cup frozen blueberries ◆ 4-6 packets of sweetener ◆ 1 teaspoon alcohol-free, sugar-free extract (vanilla, strawberry, maple, etc.)

Orange, Sliced

Peel the orange or slice off the skin with a sharp knife so that the inner film of white is entirely removed. Slice quite thinly. Sprinkle with granulated sweetener and a dash of cinnamon.

Ingredients

1 orange ◆ sweetener ◆ cinnamon

Rhubarb, Baked

Peel and cut rhubarb in 3- or 4-inch stalks. Arrange rhubarb in 1 1/2-quart casserole dish with a cover. Add water, sweetener, and salt. Measure & serve.

Ingredients

1 1/2 pounds rhubarb ◆ 1/4 cup water ◆ sweetener ◆ dash of salt

Strawberry-Rhubarb-Apple Compote

In a single microwavable bowl (if microwaving) or saucepan (if cooking on stove) Clean and pare the strawberries. Peel and core and cut up the apples. Slice the rhubarb in 1/2-1" pieces or open frozen rhubarb and place in bowl or saucepan. Combine all ingredients If Microwaving: Cook 10 minutes on Power 8 or Power High. If Cooking on Stove: Cook 25 minutes at slow simmer covered. When all ingredients are cooked to a stew, stir to blend. Let cool. When ingredients are cooled, measure 1 cup portion or 8 oz portion (depending if you cup or weigh your food.) Put portions in plastic or glass containers, leaving some room at the top for expansion in the freezer. Freeze for future use. Makes about 5 Cups. Microwave to thaw. Measure portion.

Ingredients

1 pint strawberries ◆ 5 apples (Rome apples or Rome, Fiji & GrannySmith best) ◆ 3 stalks fresh rhubarb or 1 12-16 oz. pkg frozen rhubarb

Fruit with Protein

Apple Nut Breakfast

Blend cheese, sweetener, and extract with hand mixer, until smooth. Spoon over apple and top with soy nuts before serving.

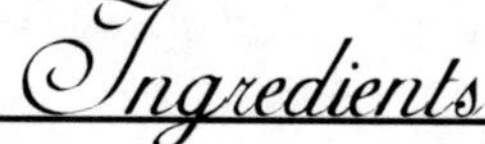

3/8 cup ricotta cheese ◆ 1 ounce roasted split soy nuts ◆ 1 apple ◆ chocolate extract ◆ sweetener

Apple Pie for Breakfast!

In a mini food processor, process 2oz of soy flour with enough water to form a soft dough and the dough gathers into ball. Press the dough into the bottom and up the sides of a small Pyrex dish sprayed with Pam. Chop 1 apple coarsely in the food processor and season with cinnamon, nutmeg and cloves and sweetener...I use Stevia (1dropperful). Place the apples on top of the prepared crust. Grind together 1oz.TVP, 1oz. Soy nuts, 1oz. soy flour to consistency of crumb topping. Flavor with sweetener and any type of flavoring you might like that is alcohol free. I used Frontier's butter flavor. Spread the crumb topping on top of the apples. Cook for 8 minutes! Measure and serve.

Ingredients

1 Apple ◆ 3 oz Soy flour ◆ Cinnamon ◆ Nutmeg ◆ Cloves ◆ Sweetener ◆ 1oz.TVP ◆ 1oz. Soy nuts

Apple Shake

Put all ingredients in blender except apples, and blend to mix. Then add the frozen apples.

Ingredients

8 oz. milk ◆ 8 oz. frozen apples ◆ apple pie spice (check to make sure NO sugar) ◆ vanilla flavoring ◆ sweetener if desired

Breakfast

This makes an excellent finger food breakfast that I can eat "on the go" while I am working.

Ingredients

1 apple sliced thin
◆ 2 oz cooked bacon strips cold and cut in to quarters
◆ 1 oz thinly sliced sharp cheddar cheese

Breakfast

This makes an excellent finger food breakfast that I can eat "on the go" while I am working.

Ingredients

Any one fruit choice from the GS ◆ 1 egg ◆ 1 oz cooked bacon strips
◆ 1/2 of it crumbled ◆ 1/2 left in strips ◆ 1/2 oz cheese
◆ 2T salsa (check with sponsor)

Breakfast

Mix together.

Ingredients

1/2 cup ricotta cheese ◆ 1/2 cup blueberries ◆ 1 packet sweetener

Breakfast Combo

Mix the peaches and yogurt together in a small serving bowl. In another bowl, mix together the soy cake ingredients. Pour the soy cake mix into a small flat bottom pan sprayed with non stick. Microwave for 3-4 minutes until the cake is formed. Slide it on to your yogurt and fruit mixture. Top with extra sweetener.

Ingredients

8oz peaches (or any other fruit you like) ◆ 6oz yogurt ◆ Soy cake:1oz soyflour with 1/4 cup diet soda or club soda ◆ sweetener (if so desired) ◆ artificial flavoring

Breakfast Muffin

Mix all ingredients together to make batter. Bake in large muffin tins for approx. 30 minutes at 350 degrees

Ingredients

1 Egg ◆ 1 oz. Soy Flour ◆ 1/2 oz. Cheese (any variety) ◆ Stevia for sweetening ◆ 1 cup. Fruit (I've used pineapple, apple, & cranberry, but it's your choice) ◆ Frontier Flavorings (or Bickford Flavors) of your choice

Dreamsicle

Blend all ingredients in food processor. Freeze overnight

Ingredients

1 cup low fat yogurt ◆ peeled and quartered orange ◆ vanilla flavoring ◆ artificial sweetener

Cranberry Orange Soy Loaf

Grind texturized soy protein into a powder, using a nut grinder or coffee grinder. Mix all ingredients, and spread in large, square, microwavable dish sprayed with Pam. Cook approximately 3 minutes loosely covered until set. Heat it before serving, and top it with zero-calorie butter spray.

Ingredients

2 ounces ground texturized soy protein ◆ 1 egg ◆ 1/2 cup cranberries ◆ 1/4 teaspoon unsweetened Orange kool-aid ◆ 3/8 cup water ◆ zero-calorie butter spray sweetener

Creamy Fruit Topping

Beat egg and pour into heated saute pan (like making an omelet) on med-low heat. Allow egg to cook until no longer soupy, then flip the entire egg patty and cook other side. In separate bowl, mix cheese, fruit & sweetener together. Spoon cheese mixture on top of egg patty.

Ingredients

1 egg ◆ 1/4 cup (1 oz.) ricotta or cottage cheese ◆ 1 serving of fruit ◆ sweetener to taste

Dutch Apple Omelet

Whip together eggs, water and first three spices. Vegetable spray the fry pan. Heat pan. Pour egg/spice mixture into pan. Cook as you would any omelet. Optional: Cover pan. (Covering the pan while cooking will expedite the cooking time.) When the egg mixture is 1/2 or 3/4th done, add apple and cover again. Cook until the apple juice has just about evaporated and caramelized. Uncover the pan for a minute or two. Turn onto a plate. Garnish plate and omelet with cinnamon.

Ingredients

2 eggs (warmed up to room temperature)
◆ 1 Tablespoon or so of water ◆ Allspice ◆ Nutmeg
◆ Pumpkin Pie Spice (Shilling Brand)
◆ 1 W&M Apple (Roughly chopped) ◆ Cinnamon (Garnish)

Favorite Saturday Breakfast

Pour sweetened whipped milk over fruit.

Ingredients

2 eggs ◆ 1 cup milk with 2 packets Equal whipped in ◆ 1 cup various mixed fruits OR 1/2 cantaloupe

Frozen Blueberry, Strawberry,or Pineapple Ricotta "Cheesecake"

Start with a serving of blueberries - or strawberries or crushed pineapple. The fruit can either be fresh, frozen and thawed, or canned - as long as it is the abstinent kind of course. Now add ricotta cheese. The amount is up to you - it can be most should be most of a protein portion - but you should leave either a half ounce or an ounce of protein for the last ingredient. Now add either or both of two optional ingredients: preferred abstinent sweetener to taste, and alcohol-free vanilla extract. Combine all ingredients so far in a small, freezer-proof container, i.e. Tupperware. It is not necessary to blend or mix completely. Mixing well with a fork should be sufficient. Finally, put the container in the freezer. It usually takes about two hours in the freezer to reach the consistency I like, but you can experiment. Don't worry if you over freeze - 20-40 seconds in the microwave should fix it. The microwave method also works if you want to make several in advance and leave them in the freezer.

Ingredients

Blueberries or Strawberries or Pineapple ◆ 1/2 cup Ricotta Cheese ◆ Sweetener ◆ Vanilla Extract ◆ TVP

Fruit Cobbler with Soy Crust

Preheat oven to 450°F (or 425, if using glass dish). Slice fruit into roughly 1-inch sections, if necessary. Spread fruit over the bottom of a small baking pan. Pour the 2 Tbl. sweetener over fruit. Set the dish in hot oven while preparing topping. Combine soy granules with salt and cinnamon in a medium-sized bowl. Add egg, yogurt, vanilla, the 1 tsp. sweetener, and zero calorie butter spray. Mix with spatula until you have a ball of pastry-type dough. You shouldn't need to add more than a few tablespoons of water, if any. Drop batter by spoonfuls on top of hot fruit. Bake 20 minutes, or until lightly browned. Suggested fruit: rhubarb and strawberries, apples and strawberries, cranberries, blueberries, peaches, or apricots.

Ingredients

1 ounce finely ground texturized soy protein ◆ 1 egg ◆ 1/4 cup yogurt ◆ 1 cup fresh fruit ◆ 2 tablespoons liquid sweetener ◆ 1 teaspoon vanilla ◆ 1 teaspoon liquid sweetener or Equal to taste ◆ 1/4 teaspoon salt ◆ 1/2 teaspoon cinnamon ◆ zero-calorie butter spray

Gjetost Cheese and Apple, Baked

Cut apple in chunks. Cut cheese in small slices or chunks, and place on top of apple. Top with cinnamon and sweetener or coffee syrup. Microwave for 30 seconds or until cheese is melted.

Ingredients

2 ounces Gjetost cheese ◆ 1 apple ◆ cinnamon ◆ sweetener or sugar-free coffee syrup

Hot Apple with Ricotta Cheese

First, you need to heat the apple. If the apple is sliced, it can be heated in either an oven, a microwave, or sautéed in a small pan - in this case, either in oil, butter, or Pam. If the apple is whole, don't use the pan method. Heat the apple until warm soft. Then top with ricotta cheese, and, if desired, sweetener, vanilla extract, cinnamon, and some crunchy TVP as an additional topping. At this point, you can either eat it as it is - the contrast between the hot apple and the cold ricotta is quite nice - or you can nuke the whole thing briefly in the microwave.

Ingredients

Apple ◆ Oil/Butter/Pam ◆ Ricotta Cheese ◆ Optional: Sweetener ◆ Vanilla Extract ◆ Cinnamon ◆ Crunchy TVP

Legal Peach "Cobbler"

Put the 2 oz soy flakes in the bottom of a bowl and top with 8 oz frozen peaches. Add butter (however much you are supposed to use for your fat). Microwave 7-8 minutes until peaches are hot. Top with Splenda. The soy flakes absorb the liquid from the frozen peaches and the butter, giving the consistency of a 'crumble.'

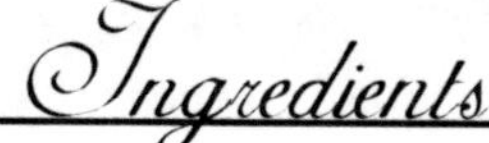

2 oz soy flakes ◆ 8 oz frozen peaches ◆ Butter ◆ Splenda to taste

Muffins

Mix well. Pour into small round rubber maid container, diameter 3 inches, and microwave on high 6 minutes. Let cook 2 minutes. Turn on to plates.

Ingredients

2 oz soy flour ◆ 2 oz fruit ◆ blueberries ◆ pineapple or apple ◆ 2 equals ◆ 3/4 tsp. Cinnamon ◆ vanilla to taste ◆ 1/2 cup diet cream soda

Orange & Ricotta

Peel and cut oranges into bite size pieces. Add ricotta, flavor with vanilla flavor (no-alcohol), one equal (not totally necessary) Yummy. Strawberries, blueberries, apple sprinkled with cinnamon- can be substituted.

Ingredients

1 Navel Orange (no seeds) ◆ 4oz Ricotta Cheese

Peach Soy Loaf

Preheat oven to 350°F, and spray a small loaf tin with Pam. Beat the egg together with the milk, cinnamon, salt, and sweetener. Whisk in the ground texturized soy protein, and beat until smooth. Fold in the peaches, pour into the baking tin. Bake for 50 minutes. Allow to cool 15 minutes before serving. I often leave these in the oven to cool overnight and dry out some of the moisture.

Ingredients

1 egg ◆ 1.5 ounces ground texturized soy protein ◆ 1/4 cup milk ◆ 1 cup peaches - chopped ◆ pinch of cinnamon ◆ dash of salt ◆ 1 tablespoon liquid or powder sweetener

Peaches and Cream

Mix ricotta cheese and frozen peaches in a blender, or food processor, and chop until fine, but not blended smooth. Stir in extract and sweetener. Top with soy nuts.

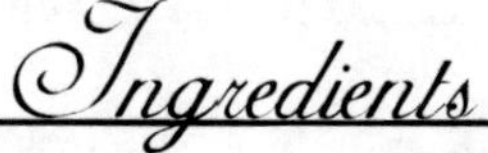

3 ounces ricotta cheese ◆ 1 ounce roasted split soy nuts ◆ 1 cup frozen peaches with no syrup added ◆ 1 tablespoon vanilla extract ◆ sweetener

Plum Crisp

Topping: To make the topping, mix coarse texturized soy protein, salt, vanilla, butter spray, sweetener, and 1 tsp. cinnamon, adding a few drops of water at a time, until the mixture resembles coarse crumbs. Stir in fine soy granules. Add additional sweetener and a few tablespoons of water, and mix until it clings together in small lumps. Set aside. Fruit Sauce: Mix together plums, sweetener, and cinnamon. Place in a small baking pan or ovenproof dish, sprayed with Pam. Sprinkle evenly with topping, and spray top with Pam for browning purposes. Bake at 350°F about 40 minutes, or until topping is brown and plums are tender.

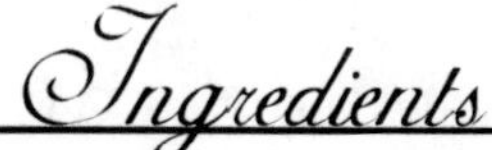

2 ounces coarsely ground texturized soy protein ◆ 2 ounces finely ground texturized soy protein ◆ 2 plums, sliced and pitted ◆ 1 tablespoon liquid sweetener or Equal to taste ◆ zero calorie butter spray ◆ 2 teaspoons cinnamon ◆ 1 tablespoon vanilla ◆ salt

Quickie breakfasts

Mix and eat with fruit.

Ingredients

3/4 cup yogurt ◆ 1 oz. soy granules (add right before eating)

Quickie breakfasts II

Cut up apples, sprinkle with cinnamon and dip in ricotta cheese. Measure portion.

Ingredients

sliced apples ◆ cinnamon ◆ ricotta cheese

Ricotta-Pineapple GS Sorbet

The night before you are ready to use take your GS pineapple, your GS Ricotta, blend in the blender. After blended, put up in a bowl or glass and freeze overnight. Ready to use in the morning.

Ingredients

1 cup Pineapple ◆ 1/2 cup Ricotta

Root Beer Moat

Peel the apple, and chop it up into 1/2-inch cubes. Put everything, except the Diet Root Beer, in a blender. Blend until smooth. Turn on frozen yogurt maker. Pour ingredients slowly into top hole of yogurt maker, while its bowl is spinning. Stop the yogurt maker when mixture thickens, and the stirrer is no longer moving. Serve immediately, or freeze for serving later. Pour desired amount of diet root beer in the serving dish. This makes 1 protein and 1 fruit. Other extract flavors and diet sodas work, too!

Ingredients

1 cup milk ◆ 1/4 cup cottage cheese or 1/2 cup plain yogurt ◆ 1 chilled apple ◆ 1 can, or bottle, of chilled diet root beer ◆ sweetener ◆ 1 tablespoon vanilla extract

Rutti Tutti Surprise

Cube sausage patties and cook in saute pan until slightly browned. Beat egg and pour into heated saute pan (like making an omelet) on medium-low heat. Allow egg to cook until no longer soupy, then flip the entire egg patty and cook other side. Once cooked, place egg patty on plate and top with sausage and cooked fruit.

Ingredients

1 egg ◆ 2 oz. breakfast sausage patties (cubed) ◆ 1 serving of fruit ◆ sweetened

Shake

Mix.I use a Braun hand blender. It comes with its own cup very convenient and I lose nothing transferring from one container to another. Taste great with frozen strawberries or frozen peaches. I use frozen fruit in no-sugar or juices. Also frozen fruit is great because the shake comes out thick and frothy.

Ingredients

4oz Yogurt ◆ 8oz Soy Milk ◆ 4oz frozen Blueberries ◆ equal ◆ Vanilla flavoring

Soy Cereal with Fruit

Just before serving, mix everything together.

Ingredients

3/4 cup milk mixed with 1 tablespoon vanilla ◆ 2 ounces granular texturized soy protein ◆ 1/2 ounce soy nuts 1 apple ◆ chopped

Soy Grit, Yogurt Porridge

Boil 1/2 cup water, and add soy grits or texturized soy protein Cook 1-2 minutes. Remove from heat. Add remaining ingredients and stir.

Ingredients

1 ounce soy grits (reconstituted finely ground texturized soy protein may be substituted) ◆ 3/4 cup yogurt ◆ 1/2 cup blueberries, or 1 apple ◆ sweetener

Soy Loaf

Preheat oven to 350°F, and spray a small loaf tin with Pam. Beat the egg together with the milk, spices, salt, and sweetener. Whisk in the ground texturized soy protein, and beat until smooth. Fold in the fruit, pour into the baking tin. Bake for 50 minutes. Allow to cool 15 minutes before serving. Leaving these in the oven to cool overnight will dry out some of the moisture. Great for traveling! May be frozen.

Ingredients

1 egg ◆ 1 1/2 ounces ground texturized soy protein ◆ 1/4 cup milk ◆ 1/2 cup cranberries or 2 plums ◆ 2 teaspoons vanilla ◆ 1 teaspoon cinnamon ◆ dash of salt ◆ sweetener

Soynut Butter Granola

Mix spices into TVP, add to softened soynut butter and mash together with fork. Mix in fruit.

Ingredients

2 oz. Protein as ◆ 1 oz. soynut butter ◆ remaining 1 oz. TVP ◆ cinnamon ◆ ground cloves (if desired) ◆ ground anise (if desired) ◆ sweetener to taste ◆ 1 fruit of your choice

Strawberries and Pineapple Tropical Delight

Measure and combine all fruit and protein in food processor. Blend until mixed well. Pour into shallow plastic dish with cover. Place in freezer for at least 4 hours. Top with coffee syrup, or extract, and sweetener. If frozen solid, place in microwave for 30 seconds, to thaw, before serving.

Ingredients

1/2 cup cottage cheese or 1 cup yogurt
◆ 1 cup mixed- 1/4 cup pineapple and 3/4 cup strawberries ◆ sweetener
◆ sugar-free Da Vinci Coconut coffee syrup Frontier Coconut extract

Strawberry Cheese Squares

Add the extract and sweetener to yogurt and stir. Chop fruit finely in food processor. Grind soy nuts into powder. In 5 X 5 dish, fold fruit into yogurt, leaving pockets. Sprinkle ground soy nuts on top, and freeze until firm. Let thaw until semi-frozen before serving.

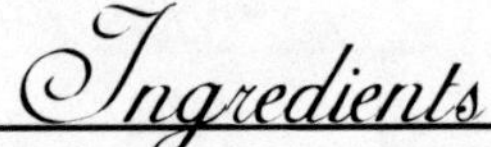

7/8 cup yogurt ◆ 1/2 ounce roasted ◆ salted soy nuts
◆ 1 cup frozen strawberries ◆ 1 1/2 tablespoons vanilla extract
◆ sweetener

The Un-Carmel Apple with soynuts

Cut up your apple lay it on a dish Pour your ghe-toast on top of the apple, add 1 oz soy nut on top of it. (I like to grind mine a bit in a coffee grinder).

Ingredients

1 apple ◆ 1 oz ghetost cheese ◆ 1oz soy nuts ◆ diet cream soda ◆ cinnamon ◆ 1-2 tsp vanilla extract ◆ 1-2 packets sweet n' low

Tofu Apple Breakfast

Crumble tofu in to a non-stick skillet that has been sprayed with non-stick spray. Stir until warm and a little brown here and there. Core apple and cut into chunks. Add cinnamon, salt, sweetener. Microwave on high for approximately 4 minutes. Combine the tofu with the apple and mix.

Ingredients

4 oz. Firm Tofu ◆ 1 apple ◆ ½ tsp. Cinnamon ◆ ¼ tsp. Celtic salt (or plain salt to taste) ◆ Sweeten to taste - artificial sweetener or stevia

Warm and Hearty Breakfast

Sprinkle apple with cinnamon and bake in microwave for 3-5 minutes. Soak soy granules in water to soften them. (Pour just enough water to cover them, and depending on how quickly the water is absorbed, you may add a little more water.) Cut cheese into tiny chunks. Scramble egg and cheese into soy granules. Add apple into the mixture, and cook in microwave for another 3 minutes, or until the egg is no longer runny.

Ingredients

1 ounce texturized soy protein ◆ 1 egg ◆ 1/2 ounce Gjetost cheese ◆ 1 chopped apple ◆ cinnamon, and sweetener

Warm Cereal with Fruit

Microwave for 2 to 3 minutes or until mixture is no longer gelatinous.

Ingredients

2 oz. TVP ◆ 1 egg ◆ 4 to 8 oz. fruit(s) of choice ◆ sweetener (if desired), cinnamon (sprinkled)

Cooked Vegetable

3 ingredient easy main course for the tired at night

Weigh & measure mushrooms & sauce according to your sponsor. Cook the big mushroom caps in tomato sauce for about 1/2 hour, letting them simmer so they get soft. Top with 1 ounce of grated cheese. Measure portions.

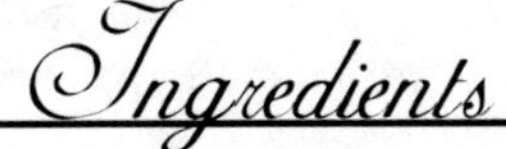

Portabella Mushroom caps ◆ your favorite tomato sauce ◆ 1 ounce grated cheese

Acorn Squash

Cut 1 whole squash in half. Cook 6 minutes on medium power in microwave. Scoop out to measure 4 ozs or 1/2 cup. Top with butterscotch flavoring.

Ingredients

1 acorn squash ◆ butterscotch flavoring

Acorn Squash Puree

Put in the blender blend until soupy and you can heat up or serve cold. You could also do this with carrots and onions mixed.

Ingredients

4oz Squash ◆ Cinnamon ◆ Vanilla flavoring ◆ Water

Acorn/Winter Squash

Cut them in half, remove the seeds, (save to plant) sprinkle cinnamon and sweetener (and extracts if you like per previous recipe) inside the hollowed out space. Then turn upside down and bake them in a 375 oven on a sprayed pan. The skins on. The skins get shinny and pretty. They take a good long while, 45 minutes or more. Should be tender when pierced with toothpick or the like.You can then scrape out the yellow meat, weight and measure and put back into the shell if you like.

Ingredients

Acorn or Winter Squash

Artichoke, Baked

Cut off bottom and about one inch off the tops of the artichoke. Rinse thoroughly. Slice artichoke lengthwise into eighths. Place into a baking pan. Spray with zero-calorie butter spray, and sprinkle seasonings over them. Spread slices out on bottom of pan. Overlapping is ok. Cover the pan with foil and bake in a 350 Fahrenheit oven for 40 min. Take foil off, mix them up and continue baking for 5 more min. Measure 1 cup and serve.

Ingredients

1 artichoke ◆ zero-calorie butter spray (olive oil flavor is good) ◆ dry basil ◆ dry oregano ◆ cayenne ◆ salt

Artichokes, Boiled or Steamed

Tear off coarse outside leaves. Cut the stem, so that the fond (bottom) will rest flat on a plate. Trim the top by slicing off 1 1/2 to 1 3/4 inches with a knife. Wash the artichoke under running water. Place artichoke in a deep kettle with salt and lemon juice. Add boiling water to cover, or steam with salt, lemon juice, and very little water. Boil or steam 30 to 45 minutes. Artichokes are done when a leaf can be easily pulled out. Remove and set upside down to drain. Measure 1 cup and serve hot or chilled. Serve hot with allowable portion of butter or chilled with allowable portion of mayonnaise.

Ingredients

1 artichoke ◆ 1 teaspoon salt ◆ 1 teaspoon lemon juice ◆ butter or mayonnaise

Artichokes, Steamed with Curry Dipping Sauce

Cut the tops and stem end off the artichoke. Steam artichoke for 45 minutes. Measure 1 cup. Mix curry powder into allowable portion of mayonnaise until it reaches the level of spiciness that suits you.

Ingredients

1 artichoke ◆ mayonnaise ◆ curry powder

Asparagus, Broiled

Wash asparagus. Trim if necessary. Place in casserole dish. Spray with zero-calorie butter spray. Place garlic slices randomly between asparagus pieces (the more garlic, the better! - minced garlic works fine also). Sprinkle lightly with salt. Broil in oven for 10-15 minutes, or until slightly browned and crispy. Measure 1 cup and serve.

Ingredients

1 - 2 bunches of asparagus
◆ zero-calorie butter spray (olive flavor is good)
◆ 2 -3 garlic cloves, thinly sliced, salt

Asparagus, Cooked

Peel stalks with a peeler. Wash thoroughly to remove sand trapped in tips and under the spurs. Place asparagus in skillet. Pour in enough cold water to cover and add salt. Bring to a boil quickly. Cook till done to your taste. Measure 1 cup. Serve hot or chilled. Serve hot with allowable portion of butter or 1/2 oz. Parmesan cheese. Serve cold with allowable portion of mayonnaise.

Ingredients

2 bunches of asparagus ◆ salt
◆ 1/2 ounce Parmesan cheese (optional) ◆ butter

Asparagus, Roasted

Heat oven to 400°F. Line a pan with aluminum foil. Rinse asparagus, and snap off tough ends. Lightly pat dry. Spread asparagus out in pan. Spray with zero-calorie butter spray, and sprinkle with salt and pepper. Mix seasonings and asparagus with spatula. Pat into a single layer. Bake until asparagus are tender and lightly crisped; about 15 minutes. Shake pan once or twice during baking time. Measure 1 cup and serve. Roasting brings out the natural sweetness in most vegetables, and intensifies their flavor.

Ingredients

1 1/2 pounds slender asparagus ◆ tough ends snapped off
◆ zero-calorie butter spray (olive oil flavored) ◆ 1 teaspoon salt
◆ 1/2 teaspoon black pepper

Baked Spanish Onion

Cut a large, sweet Spanish onion in quarters. Place in a 400-degree oven. Bake 45 minutes.

Ingredients

Large Sweet Spanish Onion

Baked Turnips and Rutabagas (Greysheet Baked Potatoes)

Peel turnips and rutabagas thoroughly and scrub them. Spray with a little butter flavored PAM and poke holes (about 6). Wrap in foil but leave an opening on top. Bake at 275 degrees for about 1.5-2.0 hours until browned and soft.

Ingredients

1/2 cup or 4 ozs. Turnips ◆ or Rutabagas

Barbecue Sauce

Mix well. Store in a container in fridge.

Ingredients

Un-Ketchup.◆ Soysauce.◆ a dash or 2 of Worcestshire, and sweeten to taste with brown sugar substitute

Bean Sprouts, How To Grow

Take a few spoonfuls of any bean sprout seed, and put them in the jar. Repeat 3-4 times: Fill about 3/4 of the way with water. Secure the cheesecloth over the top with the rubber band and shake. Drain. Fill with water and let soak overnight. For the next 3-5 days, rinse sprouts and drain once a day, leaving the jar on its side in a dark, dry place (preferably tilting the jar a little to drain excess water). When sprouts are the proper length (about 5 days or so), leave them in the sun for a few hours to develop the chlorophyll. Rinse and place in an uncovered plastic container in the fridge. Rinse every day to ensure freshness. Measure 1 cup for a serving. Preparation time is 5 days.

Ingredients

bean sprout seed ◆ jar ◆ cheesecloth ◆ rubberband

Beet Greens, Cooked

Wash the greens well several times. Place in a heavy kettle. Cover tightly. Let them wilt over medium heat. Toss with a fork several times to mix the top greens with the bottom greens. When they are just wilted and tender, remove them and drain thoroughly, then chop and drain some more. Measure 1 cup. Top with allowable portion of melted butter, lemon juice, salt, pepper, and dash of nutmeg. These are pungent and pleasing to the palate.

Ingredients

1 - 2 pounds beet greens ◆ butter ◆ 1 teaspoon lemon juice ◆ salt ◆ pepper ◆ dash of nutmeg

Beets, Cooked

Put them in a small amount of boiling water, cover tightly, and simmer slowly till they are tender to the touch of the finger. Don't pierce them with a fork until they are done. They will take from 30 to 45 minutes. Plunge the cooked beets into cold water. As soon as you can handle them, slip the skins off. Beets may also be baked in the oven at 325 degrees F for an hour. Top with allowable portion of butter. Serving ideas: Serve with roast of pork or grilled pork chops.

Ingredients

8 beets ◆ 1 teaspoon lemon juice ◆ salt ◆ pepper ◆ butter

Bell Peppers, Roasted

Over an open flame on the stove, or under a broiler, roast peppers until skins are charred on all sides. Place in a paper or plastic bag and seal bag. Let peppers steam 10 minutes. When peppers are cool enough to handle, peel, seed and cut into 1/3-inch-wide strips. Transfer to a glass dish. Spray with zero-calorie butter spray. Measure 1 cup and serve.

Ingredients

4 bell peppers whole ◆ any color, zero-calorie butter spray (olive oil flavored)

Bengali Tomatoes

Heat the oil in a wok; add cumin, mustard, fennel, and fenugreek. As soon as the mustard seeds pop, put in the red pepper. Stir once; add the tomatoes and cover immediately. Turn heat to medium. When tomatoes stop making noises, take off the lid and add salt and sweetener. Cover again, turn heat to low, and simmer 7-10 minutes.

Ingredients

2 lbs canned diced tomatoes ◆ 3 Tb mustard oil
◆ 1/2 tsp whole cumin ◆ 1/2 tsp whole mustard seed
◆ 1/2 tsp whole fennel ◆ 1/2 tsp whole fenugreek
◆ 1 dried hot red pepper ◆ 1 tsp salt ◆ 1 tsp liquid sweetener

Ben's BLT Salad

Mix in a Large bowl. Measure portion.

Ingredients

allotment of fat any mixture works- chunky blue cheese ◆ 2 oz.
Tomato product -- salsa works well
◆ 1 oz. Sesame Seeds (check with your sponsor on this)
◆ 4 oz. Bacon and Soy Nuts -- any combo ◆ 24 oz. Tomatoes
◆ Peppers -- cooked veggie of just about any variety
(I sometimes use steamed, cooled cauliflower and/or broccoli)

Broccoli w/Lemon Sauce

Cut off hard ends and remove outer leaves. Soak for 30 minutes in salted water. Place in pot of 1 pint boiling water (salted). Stalks down. Remove and drain. Chop garlic very fine and mix thru. Measure out 1 cup and add lemon and margarine.

Ingredients

Broccoli ◆ garlic, lemon juice

Broccoli, Boiled

Since broccoli florets cook more quickly than stems, peel the stalks down to the white flesh and cut into short lengths. Cook in boiling, salted water for about 5 minutes. Then, add the florets and cook another 5 minutes. Drain.

Ingredients

1 cup broccoli ◆ salt

Broccoli, Steamed

Peel heavy stems. Remove thick, woody stems. Cut into smaller bunches. Rinse. It is best to steam cook broccoli standing in upright bunches. Tie bunches together and stand up in 1 1/2 inches boiling, salted water, in saucepan. If lid will not cover saucepan, cover it with foil. Steam for 12-14 minutes, or until just tender. Drain well. Measure 1 cup and serve. Top with allowable portion of butter and seasonings. Do not overcook, or flowers will break and fall off.

Ingredients

2 pounds broccoli ◆ salt ◆ butter

Broccoli, Tangy

Heat a wok or skillet. Add the sesame oil as allowable fat to cook in vegetable, or spray wok with zero-calorie butter spray. Stir fry broccoli on a high flame for 8-10 minutes. In a small bowl mix the mustard and soy sauce till smooth. Add this sauce mixture to the broccoli. Give it a quick stir and remove from flame. Measure 1 cup and serve.

Ingredients

1 pound broccoli cut into big flowerettes ◆ 2 tablespoons mustard (preferably English mustard) ◆ 2 teaspoons soy sauce ◆ allotment of sesame oil or zero-calorie butter spray (sesame flavor is good)

Broiled Tomatoes Provencale

Preheat the broiler. Core the tomatoes and cut them in half. Arrange cut side up in a baking pan. Distribute the oil over each tomato. Sprinkle with garlic, salt, and pepper. Broil for about 5 minutes, remove from heat, and serve.

Ingredients

4 ripe tomatoes ◆ olive oil ◆ 1 Tb pressed garlic ◆ 1/2 salt, pepper

Brussels Sprouts, Steamed

Cut off the stem end and remove the outer leaves and any leaves yellowed or ravaged with wormholes. Soak sprouts in water 15 to 20 minutes before cooking. Put 1/4 inch of salted water in a heavy saucepan and bring to a boil. Add sprouts, cover tightly, and steam 5 to 10 minutes, or until just crisply tender. Do not overcook. Drain well and return to saucepan to dry out before seasoning. Sprouts may also be boiled for 5 to 15 minutes, depending on the crispness desired and size. Measure 1 cup and serve. Serve with beef, lamb, roast chicken, or roast pork.

Ingredients

1 cup or 8 ozs. Brussels Sprouts ◆ Steamed

Cabbage and Tomatoes

Chop cabbage into 1-inch pieces. Place tomatoes and spices in large pot, and cook together over low heat 5 minutes. Add cabbage, cover, and cook until cabbage wilts. Uncover, stir, raise heat to medium, and continue cooking until mixture turns brown from the spices - the longer, the better. Add melted butter after weighing. Measure 1 cup and serve.

Ingredients

1 large head cabbage ◆ 32 ounces can diced tomatoes ◆ 1 tablespoon onion powder ◆ 1/2 tablespoon five-spice powder ◆ 1/4 teaspoon ground cloves ◆ 1 tablespoon worcestershire sauce ◆ 1/2 tablespoon dry mustard ◆ ground pepper ◆ salt

Cabbage and Cauliflower with Indian Spices

Cook the cauliflower in boiling water until just tender, about 3 minutes. Drain well and set aside. Heat zero-calorie cooking spray in a large, deep skillet over high heat. Add mustard seeds, coriander, cumin, and salt. When the mustard seeds begin to pop, add the onion, chili and a few tablespoons of water. Cook and stir until the onion begins to soften at the edges. Add the cabbage and cook, stirring often, until it begins to soften. Add 1 cup water and tomato paste. Reduce heat to medium, cover, and cook until cabbage is tender (about 5 minutes). Add cauliflower and lemon juice, and cook until everything is heated through. Stir in cilantro and salt to taste. Measure 1/2 cup and serve. Cilantro has a very distinctive taste; if you don't like it, leave it out.

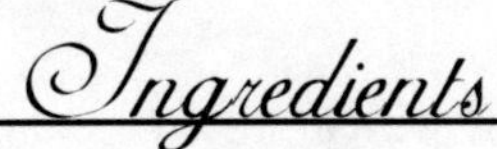

1 large head cauliflower cut into florets ◆ 1 1/2 teaspoon mustard seeds ◆ 1/2 teaspoon ground coriander ◆ 1/4 teaspoon ground cumin ◆ 1 medium onion cut into thin wedges ◆ 1 hot green chili minced ◆ 1/2 head green cabbage cut into 1-inch squares ◆ 1 tablespoon tomato paste ◆ 2 tablespoons lemon juice ◆ 1/3 cup chopped fresh cilantro ◆ salt ◆ zero-calorie cooking spray

Butternut Squash

Slice 2 whole washed butternut squashes in half the long way. Place all four halves, sliced-side-down on a cookie sheet. Bake at 400 degrees for 20 minutes, or until the skin is crispy, and the sliced sides are caramelized. Measure 1/2 cup or 4 ozs. portion.

Ingredients

Butternut Squash

Cabbage on Tomato Sauce

Put all ingredients in a plastic lunch container. To avoid marinating, do NOT mix together until serving! When ready, mix and microwave 5 - 7 minutes, depending on how crunchy you like your cabbage.

Ingredients

1/2 cup cabbage ◆ cleaned and chopped coarsely ◆ 1/2 cup chopped roma tomatoes ◆ 2 ounces tomato sauce ◆ basil

Cabbage, Boiled

Remove outer leaves which are coarse and torn. Trim the stalk. Cut the cabbage in half and cut each half in 2 or 3 sections. Or shred the cabbage very fine with a sharp knife or shredder, removing the stem. Soak for 1/2 hour in cold water with a touch of salt. Drain. Use a pot deep enough to cover cabbage in salted water. Bring water to a boil. Add cabbage. Boil over high heat, uncovered, for 8 to 10 minutes, or until just crisply tender. Drain it well. Measure 1 cup and serve.

Ingredients

1 head cabbage ◆ salt

Cabbage, Steamed

Remove outer leaves which are coarse and torn. Trim the stalk. Cut the cabbage in half and cut each half in 2 or 3 sections. Or shred the cabbage very fine with a sharp knife or shredder, removing the stem. Soak for 1/2 hour in cold water with a touch of salt. Drain. Put 1/2 inch salted water in saucepan or skillet with a tight lid. Bring water to a boil, covered. When it begins to steam, add the cabbage. Cover tightly, and reduce heat. Steam for 4 - 8 minutes. Shake the pan vigorously several times during cooking. When the cabbage is just crisply tender, drain it well. Measure 1 cup and serve.

Ingredients

1 head cabbage ◆ salt

Cabbage, Boiled

Remove outer leaves which are coarse and torn. Trim the stalk. Cut the cabbage in half and cut each half in 2 or 3 sections. Or shred the cabbage very fine with a sharp knife or shredder, removing the stem. Soak for 1/2 hour in cold water with a touch of salt. Drain. Use a pot deep enough to cover cabbage in salted water. Bring water to a boil. Add cabbage. Boil over high heat, uncovered, for 8 to 10 minutes, or until just crisply tender. Drain it well. Measure 1 cup and serve.

Ingredients

1 head cabbage ◆ salt

Carrots, Steamed

Scrub and brush carrots clean. If carrots are old, scrape or peel them. Cut carrots into julienned sticks, shred, or keep whole. Heat a very small amount of salted water in a heavy saucepan with a tight-fitting cover. Drop in the carrots. Cover, and steam gently until tender. Steam 3 - 4 minutes, if shredded. Steam 10 - 12 minutes, if cut. Steam 15 - 18 minutes, if whole. Measure 1/2 cup and serve. Serving ideas: Top with allowable portion of butter, lemon juice, marjoram, fresh dill, and/or parsley.

Ingredients

2 to 8 carrots ◆ depending on the size ◆ salt

Cauliflower with Indian Spices

In a large skillet, melt allowable portion of 1/2 butter and 1/2 oil over medium heat. Add cumin, coriander, and ginger. Cook spices until fragrant, about one minute. Add tomato and cauliflower florets to skillet. Gently mix until cauliflower is evenly coated with spice mixture. Add 1/4 cup water. Cover; cook 20 minutes, until cauliflower is tender. Season with salt and pepper. Measure 1 cup and serve.

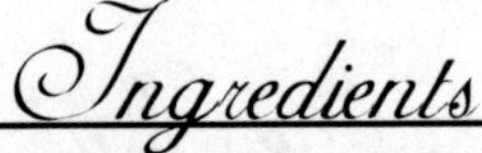

1 medium head cauliflower separated into small florets ◆ 1 small tomato, finely chopped ◆ part butter, part canola oil ◆ 1 teaspoon ground cumin ◆ 1/2 teaspoon ground coriander ◆ 1/2 teaspoon ground ginger ◆ salt and pepper

Cauliflower, Roasted

Preheat oven to 500 degrees F. Spray flat pan with zero-calorie butter spray. Add cauliflower with seasonings. Roast in middle of oven for 12 to 15 minutes, until browned in spots and tender. Measure 1 cup and serve.

Ingredients

1 head cauliflower, broken into florets
◆ zero-calorie butter spray (olive flavor is good)
◆ 1 teaspoon dried rosemary, crumbled ◆ salt and pepper

Cauliflower, Steamed

Wash cauliflower well. Remove outer leaves, heavy stem, and any bruised sections. Leave whole or break into flowerets. Steam in 1 inch of boiling, salted water in a heavy covered saucepan. Steam flowerets for 8 - 15 minutes. Steam whole cauliflower 20 - 30 minutes. Drain thoroughly. Measure 1 cup and serve. Serving ideas: Top with allowable portion of butter, Gruyere cheese, shredded cheddar cheese, grated Parmesan cheese, chives and parsley, pepper, and/or paprika.

Ingredients

1 head cauliflower ◆ salt

Cauliflower-Onion Mashed

Steam or nuke the cauliflower and onions. Puree the cauliflower until creamy smooth. Spray with "I cant believe its not butter" spray and stir/add in onions. Put into a large baking pan and sprinkle with paprika. Bake until it is browned on top.

Ingredients

1 cup or 8 ozs. Cauliflower ◆ 1/4 cup Onions ◆ Paprika

Celery Cabbage, Fried

Wash the cabbage and shred finely. Wash the celery and cut into thin slices. Spray pan with zero-calorie spray. Fry the cabbage for 3 minutes, stirring all the time. Add the salt, mixing well. Add celery to the cabbage with 2 tablespoons water. Cook over a fierce heat, stirring all the time, for 2 minutes.

Ingredients

1 pound white or Chinese cabbage ◆ 2 sticks celery, sliced thin ◆ zero-calorie butter spray ◆ 1 teaspoon salt

Chinese Eggplant

Put a small amount of peanut oil or sesame oil in a small frying pan and add chopped garlic, grated fresh ginger, and soy sauce. Toss the eggplant in the frying pan.

Ingredients

Eggplant, cut in 1" chunks and steamed till soft ◆ chopped garlic ◆ grated fresh ginger ◆ soy sauce

Chinese Turnip Stew

Heat the oil in a heavy-bottomed pot over medium flame. Add garlic and ginger; stir and fry for 15 seconds. Add turnips, green beans, and carrots; stir and fry for 1 minute. Add mushrooms and stir for another minute. Put in 2 cups water, soy sauce, vinegar, and sweetener. Bring to a boil. Cover, lower heat, and simmer for about 20 minutes or until turnips are just tender. Remove cover and turn heat to high. Boil away most of the liquid.

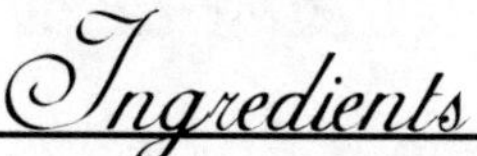

allotment of olive oil ◆ 2 cloves garlic peeled and lightly crushed ◆ 2 quarter-sized slices of fresh ginger ditto ◆ 1 lb turnips peeled and cut into 1 1/2-inch cubes ◆ 1/2 lb green beans cut into 2-inch lengths ◆ 2 carrots peeled and cut crosswise into 1 1/2-inch lengths ◆ 6 oz mushrooms washed and trimmed ◆ 2 Tb soy sauce ◆ 1 Tb vinegar ◆ 1 Tb sweetener

Cold Mediterranean Roasted Eggplant Salad

Roast eggplants in the broiler or on grill. Cut into cubes and add remaining ingredients (per 4 oz portion).

Ingredients

Eggplant ◆ 1 small clove garlic ◆ salt to taste ◆ allotment of olive oil ◆ 1 teaspoon lemon juice

Collard Greens, Braised

Spray skillet with zero-calorie butter spray. Sauté garlic over med-hi heat. When tender, add greens. Stir for 2-3 minutes, then add enough water to almost cover the greens. Stir occasionally. When greens are tender and bright green, and some of the water has boiled off, add a splash of balsamic vinegar and pepper. Measure 1 cup and serve. Variation: Also sauté with 1 medium yellow onion, on maintenance, or cut portion in half.

Ingredients

1 lb. collard greens, washed, torn, and w/ stems removed ◆ 2 large cloves garlic, minced ◆ zero-calorie butter spray (olive flavor is good) ◆ balsamic vinegar ◆ pepper

Colombo De Giraumon (Spicy Pumpkin)

Heat the oil in a heavy pan and then add the onion. Sauté until transparent and then add the garlic and hot pepper. Next put in the pumpkin, curry powder, ground cloves, the chopped tomatoes, and the sweetener. Add lemon juice. Cover and cook very gently for 30-40 minutes or until pumpkin is tender, stirring frequently to ensure that it does not stick.

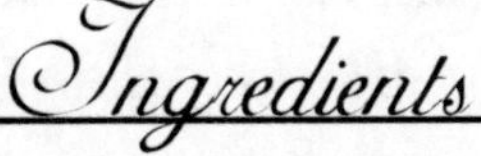

1 Onion finely sliced ◆ 2 Tomatoes chopped ◆ 1 clove Garlic pressed, ◆ 2 teaspoons Curry Powder ◆ 1 teaspoon Liquid Sweetener ◆ 1/4 teaspoon ground Cloves ◆ 2 tablespoons Lemon Juice ◆ 1/2 fresh Red Chili Pepper finely chopped ◆ allotment of Oil ◆ 1 lb Pumpkin peeled cut into 1-In. cubes ◆ Salt and Pepper

Cook and Store Beets

Rinse off the beets, put in a large pot and cover them with water. Boil for about 45 minutes. Put the pot in the sink and run cold water into it. (Wear rubber gloves to avoid staining your hands.) Let the tap run a thin stream of cold water while you slip the skin off each beet by squeezing it gently and moving it around with your thumb - the skin sort of wiggles off. Slice or dice the peeled, boiled beets. Put beets in a large covered glass dish and cover them with vinegar. Refrigerate.Measure portion.

Ingredients

beets ◆ vinegar ◆ glass container

Deep fried Spinach

Remove Spinach stems. Deep fry in oil just until crispy. Remove onto paper towel. Sprinkle with Salt.

Ingredients

1 cup or 8 ozs. Spinach ◆ allotment of. oil

Eggplant basic, grilled effect

Slice eggplant with skin in tact, about 1/4", sort of thin, but not paper thin, and definitely not fat/thick. Spread sort of in rows overlapping just a bit, but not too much, on a sprayed baking sheet. Do not overcrowd, so that each gets crispy. Set the oven for 425 degrees. I salt with McCormicks Montreal steak seasoning, dry oregano, and just a sprinkle of Sweet and low. I use the spices heavily, but that is not required. Bake in oven a long time. Test after 20 or 25 minutes to see if they look dark enough, cooked enough, or crispy enough for you. Cook time varies due to temp, and thickness of slices, could be up to 45 minutes.

Ingredients

Eggplant ◆ McCormicks Montreal Steak Seasoning ◆ Oregano ◆ Sweet-n-Low

Eggplant Dip for Raws

Cut up ripe Japanese eggplants, about 4-5 (it is sweeter than regular) Put into clear plastic produce bag and poke a hole in it and nuke for about 8 minutes until mushy. Put into the food processor with garlic powder, onion powder, salt and pepper to taste, lemon juice **check with sponsor-IF ALLOWED ON YOUR FOOD PLAN salsa **check with your sponsor Also, cook cauliflower and broccoli same way in the bag and nuke until mushy. Put all veggies into the food processor and make babaganush mush. Weigh out 8 oz and use for a dip.

Ingredients

4-5 Japanese Eggplants ◆ Cauliflower ◆ Broccoli ◆ Garlic Powder ◆ Onion Powder ◆ Salt and Pepper to taste ◆ Lemon Juice

Eggplant Easy Bake

Peel the eggplant and cut into one inch cubes. Cut the green pepper into one inch chunks. Open cans of tomatoes and cut the tomatoes in half. Combine all the cut vegetables and put into a 9-by 13-inch rectangle oven-proof pan. Add tomatoes, salt, and pepper and mix. Cover with aluminum foil and bake at 375 degrees oven for one hour. Measure 1 cup and serve. Variation: Also add 1 large sliced onion and measure 1/2 cup serving.

Ingredients

1 large egg plant ◆ 1 green pepper ◆ 2 12-ounce cans of whole tomatoes ◆ salt ◆ pepper ◆ 2 medium zucchini (optional)

Eggplant Rattouille

Season all of the veggies with oregano or any Italian seasoning, salt and pepper I take the eggplant slice it into quarters, spray a cookie sheet with Pam. Bake in oven until it begins to get tender. In the meantime cut up remaining vegetables and sauté them in a large pot sprayed with Pam. Once they are tender mix them with the eggplant and can of crusted tomatoes. Put the mixture into a casserole dish and bake until the tomatoes began to bubble and all of the veggies are tender. You can measure out 8 oz of veggies for lunch or your required amount for dinner.

Ingredients

2 Eggplant ◆ 2 Yellow squash ◆ 2 Zucchini ◆ 1 Green pepper ◆ 1 Red pepper ◆ 1 Onion ◆ 2 cloves Garlic ◆ 1 can of crushed Tomatoes ◆ Oregano ◆ Salt ◆ Ground pepper

Eggplant, Baked Puree

Heat oven to 425° F. Cut the eggplant on all sides with deep slashes and place in a baking pan. Roast until soft, 30 to 40 minutes. Set aside until cool enough to handle, about 15 minutes. Peel eggplant and coarsely chop. Place in a medium bowl. Spray with olive oil-flavored butter spray. Add garlic, salt, pepper and parsley. Measure 1 cup and serve.

Ingredients

1 eggplant or 2 Italian eggplants ◆ zero-calorie butter spray (olive oil flavor) ◆ 2 garlic cloves, pushed through a press ◆ 1/2 teaspoon salt , freshly ground black pepper to taste ◆ chopped fresh parsley to taste

Eggplant Slices

Leaving skin on, slice uniformly and lay out on sprayed cookie sheet type pan. Dot with sweetener, and heavy sprinkle with oregano. Bake well till browned at 400. Time depends on thickness of your slices. I keep them medium. Weigh out--you get a lot for 8 oz. Or if split up can be used for dipping like chips. Travel well.

Ingredients

Eggplant

Eggplant, Broiled

Peel eggplant, if desired. Cut in wedges. Place on squares of foil. Spray with zero-calorie butter spray. Sprinkle with salt, pepper, and fresh basil. Fold foil like an envelope and cook on the broiler, turning several times for 20 minutes. Or cook in oven for same amount of time. They do not need to be peeled or soaked before cooking.

Ingredients

1 eggplant ◆ zero-calorie butter spray

Eggplant

Wash an eggplant. Place in microwave either inside of plastic bag or cover with microwave cover and microwave on HI for 3 minutes. Then slice into 3/4" slices. (Not thinner they will fall apart). Spice and salt as you like. Garlic, Italian spices, Cajun spices, curry. Use your imagination. Spray frying pan with PAM or other such spray. Fry on both sides till done. Measure portion.

Ingredients

Eggplant ◆ Spices to taste

Eggplant-Spinach Curry

Heat the oil with half of the mustard seeds in a large saucepan. Add remaining mustard seeds when the cooked seeds begin to pop. Add the garlic and sauté over fairly low heat until it begins to turn golden. Add the spinach, a small amount at a time, stirring occasionally to keep it from scorching. (There is less danger of this with frozen spinach, which tends to have quite a bit of water in it.) When the spinach wilts, add the eggplant, ginger, jalapeno pepper, turmeric, paprika, coriander, and cumin. Sauté to blend the flavors. Cover and cook over medium-low heat for 15 minutes. Add the tomatoes and season to taste with salt. Cook, uncovered, 5 minutes longer. Garnish with cilantro.

Ingredients

allotment of oil ◆ 1 teaspoon black mustard seeds ◆ 12 cloves garlic peeled and coarsely chopped ◆ 2 lbs fresh spinach rinsed dried and finely chopped, (or 1 good-sized package frozen chopped spinach) ◆ 1 medium eggplant cut into 1/2-inch cubes ◆ 1-inch piece fresh ginger peeled and grated ◆ 1 jalapeno pepper minced ◆ 1/4 teaspoon turmeric ◆ 1/4 teaspoon paprika ◆ 1/2 teaspoon ground coriander ◆ 1/2 teaspoon ground cumin ◆ 1 can chopped tomatoes ◆ salt ◆ cilantro sprigs for garnish

Eksta Ginger Pumpkin Pudding

Melt butter or margarine with spices in a saucepan. Measure the pumpkin and put in a small-medium bowl. Pour the melted fat and spices over and blend well. Keep the mixture in a bowl and refrigerate. Or heat the weighed and measured 1/2 cup Ginger Pumpkin Pudding and have heated for lunch.

Ingredients

allotment of Butter or Margarine ◆ 1/2 cup Pumpkin ◆ 1 teaspoon ground Cinnamon ◆ 1 teaspoon ground Cardamom ◆ 1 teaspoon ground Cloves ◆ 1 teaspoon ground Ginger (optional) ◆ 1 teaspoon Stevia ◆ Equal or Sweet & Low

Fauxtatoe Salad

Melt butter or margarine with spices in a saucepan. Measure the pumpkin and put in a small-medium bowl. Pour the melted fat and spices over and blend well. Keep the mixture in a bowl and refrigerate. Or heat the weighed and measured 1/2 cup Ginger Pumpkin Pudding and have heated for lunch.

Ingredients

Head of cauliflower ◆ 1 oz. chopped green pepper ◆ 1 oz. chopped celery ◆ allotment of mayonnaise ◆ yellow mustard ◆ salt ◆ pepper

French Fried Turnips

Microwave the turnip for about 10 minutes. Slice the turnip into thin pieces and fry in abstinently measured olive oil or butter. (1/2 c. if rutebega; 1 c if white turnip). Measure & serve.

Ingredients

1/2 cup turnips ◆ allotment of olive oil

French Onions

Heat a large casserole or heavy pot and coat with the oil. Add onions, cover, and simmer over low heat for 2 to 3 hours, stirring thoroughly once every 10 minutes. When onions are a rich brown and very soft, mix in the butter and soy sauce and simmer 10 to 15 minutes more. For best flavor, allow to cool overnight and reheat. Measure and serve.

Ingredients

2 teaspoons Vegetable Oil ◆ 6 medium Onions sliced very thin ◆ 2 tablespoons Soy sauce ◆ allotment of Butter

Fresh Pumpkin and Rutabaga

Boil together equal parts of peeled rutabaga and pumpkin until very soft. While they are boiling, sauté onion in butter. Drain rutabaga and pumpkin and combine with onion in a large bowl; mash all until creamy and season with salt and pepper. (If you've got a big enough food-processor, mash it in there and save yourself some work.)

Ingredients

Equal parts peeled fresh pumpkin and peeled rutabaga ◆ cut into chunks ◆ 1 onion, finely chopped ◆ allotment of butter ◆ salt and pepper

Golden Rutabaga - Double Cooked-Baked

Take 1 yellow rutebaga. Slice round slices and then slice these into 1/2 to 3/4 in strips. Cook the strips in a microwave on high for about 8 minutes or boil the strips in water until very tender. Take the cooked strips and place in a baking pan or dish. Brush 1 tablespoon oil on strips. Place baking dish in oven at 350 degrees. Bake about 20 minutes until "beautifully golden". (1/2 c. abstinent amount) Measure and serve

Ingredients

rutabaga ◆ allotment of butter or oil

Green Beans

Get a few packages of frozen green beans and spread them out on aluminum foil (perhaps on top of cookie sheets) and bake them until they're crisp. Weighed they're supposed to give you a LOT. Sprinkle with abstinent butter salt (back years ago I used Durkee's) and if you want, eat them with abstinent ketchup, contingent, of course, on sponsor approval.

Ingredients

Frozen green beans

Greens, Cooked

Wash greens with several waters, dry them, and wash again. Discard any brown or faded leaves. What water remains on the greens after the washing is enough for their cooking. Place the greens and salt in a heavy saucepan with a tight-fitting cover. Let them wilt over medium heat. For collards, cook 10 - 15 minutes. For mustard and chard, cook 15 - 18 minutes. For turnip greens, cook 15 - 25 minutes. Drain them well. Chop, if desired. Serving ideas: Top with allowable portion of butter, lemon juice, and/or pork or ham. Measure and serve.

Ingredients

1 - 2 pounds collard greens ◆ mustard greens ◆ turnip greens and/or chard ◆ salt

Grilled Carrots

Spray baby carrots with Pam butter spray and sprinkle with Splenda and cinnamon. Cook for about 40-45 minutes on low grill heat (farthest rack from the fire) until soft and start getting browned (semi-burned). Measure and serve.

Ingredients

Baby carrots ◆ Pam butter spray ◆ Splenda ◆ cinnamon

Grilled Cipolline Onions

Preheat broiler or grill. If you are using wooden skewers, soak them in water. Measure the oil into a small bowl. Peel onions and cut off both ends. If the onions are more than 1-inch thick, slice them in half. Thread onto skewers. Brush with the oil until thoroughly covered, then sprinkle with salt and pepper.

Ingredients

1-2 lbs cipolline onions ◆ allotment of good Italian olive oil ◆ salt and pepper

Grilled Vegetable Medley

Chop all vegetables. Toss with spices, soy sauce, vinegar and water, or just 1 cup water. Cook in microwave 5 minutes on high. Transfer mixture to a wire grill and place on barbecue. Baste with reserved soy-water mixture. Grill for 10 to 15 minutes, turning occasionally. Measure 1 cup and serve. Variation: Also use 1 large spanish onion, cut into 8 to 12 chunks, and measure 1/2 cup serving.

Ingredients

1 each green and red bell peppers, in large chunks ◆ 1/2 pound whole button mushrooms ◆ 2 stalks celery, in 1 1/2-inch pieces ◆ 12 whole cherry tomatoes ◆ 1 small zucchini, sliced 1/2-inch thick ◆ 2 tablespoons soy sauce ◆ 1/2 cup vinegar, if allowed ◆ 1/2 cup water ◆ dashes of pepper ◆ parsley ◆ oregano ◆ basil

Harvard GS Beets

Combine ingredients, heat and serve. Heat and serve.

Ingredients

1/2 cup canned beets ◆ sweetener ◆ allspice ◆ cloves ◆ nutmeg

Indian "Dry" Turnips

Boil the turnips at least 4 hours in advance of cooking. (You can leave them overnight.) When you're ready to begin, peel the boiled turnips and dice into pieces about 1 inch x 1/2-inch. Boil the turnips at least 4 hours in advance of cooking. (You can leave them overnight.) When you're ready to begin, peel the boiled turnips and dice into pieces about 1 inch x 1/2-inch.

Ingredients

1 lb turnips ◆ 3 tsp vegetable oil ◆ 1/8 tsp asafetida ◆ 1 tsp whole fennel seeds ◆ 1 tsp whole cumin seeds ◆ 1 tsp whole black mustard seeds ◆ 12 whole fenugreek seeds ◆ 3 whole dried hot red peppers ◆ 1/2 tsp ground turmeric ◆ 1 1/2 tsp salt ◆ 1 Tb lemon juice

Italian Green Peppers & Onions

Put peppers and onions in a deep frying pan with olive oil. Cook on high for 5 minutes to brown lightly. Turn heat down. Cover and cook 20 minutes, tossing lightly.

Ingredients

2 to 3 cups cut up green peppers and onions ◆ allotment of olive oil

Japanese Lemon Squash

Peel squash and cut into 2-inch cubes. Combine squash, 1 1/4 cups water, sweetener, salt, and soy sauce in a saucepan. Cover with drop-lid or plate, then pan lid. Simmer until squash is tender and liquid nearly absorbed. Turn off heat, uncover, add lemon juice, and replace pan lid. Allow to stand 3 or 4 minutes to let lemon flavor blend in.

Ingredients

2 1/2 lbs winter squash ◆ 4 tablespoon liquid sweetener ◆ 1/2 teaspoon salt ◆ 2 tablespoon soy sauce ◆ 1 tablespoon lemon juice

Kabocha Heaven

Get a ripe Kabocha squash (it is dark green outside and orange inside, shaped like a pumpkin). Poke a few holes and bake at 375 for about 1 1/2 hours until mushy inside.

Ingredients

Kabocha Squash

Lemon Ginger Pumpkin

Finely grate the lemon. Measure the pumpkin in a bowl. Mix in lemon peel, sweetener, ginger. Bake in the middle of the oven at 350 degrees for 10 - 12 minutes. Or Microwave for 1-2 minutes. Allow to cool slightly. Or the Lemon Ginger Pumpkin may be refrigerated and eaten cold.

Ingredients

Grated Peel from 1/2 lemon ◆ 1 teaspoon ground Ginger ◆ 1 teaspoon scant Equal ◆ Stevia ◆ Sweet 'n Low ◆ 1/2 cup Pumpkin Puree

Mixed Root Vegetable Puree

Measure vegetables cooked. Mash all vegetables together with a mixer to remove lumps. Mix in seasonings. Measure 1/2 cup and serve hot. Top with allowable portion of butter and/or zero-calorie butter spray, if desired.

Ingredients

16 ounces cooked carrots ◆ 16 ounces cooked rutabagas ◆ 2 cans cooked pumpkin ◆ 1/2 to 1 teaspoon nutmeg ◆ sweetener to taste ◆ salt (optional)

Mashed Butternut Squash

Seed and quarter squash. Method I: Pressure Cooker–Place the cooking rack in the pressure cooker in order to keep the squash out of the liquid. Add the water. Place the squash on the rack. Close the cover securely. Place the pressure regulator on the vent. Cook at 15 POUNDS for 8 minutes (start timing when the regulator begins to rock). Immerse the pressure cooker in or under running cold water to stop the cooking. Remove the squash. Remove the rack. Discard the remaining water. Cool the squash. Remove and discard the skin. Mash the squash with the sweetener, butter, vinegar and mustard. Season to taste salt and pepper. Return to the pressure cooker. Cook over medium heat until hot. Serve. Method II: Microwave- Place squash onplate and microwave for 2 minutes on high. Remove squash from microwave. Slice off top and bottom and cut into large chunks, removing seeds from bottom portion. Place in a microwave-proof container with about 1/2 inch of water, cover and microwave on high until squash is extremely soft. Peel away the skin (mind your fingers!) and place squash in a large mixing bowl. Mash the squash and beat it together with the sweetener, butter, vinegar and mustard. Season to taste with salt and pepper. Reheat in microwave before serving.

Ingredients

1 1/2 cups water ◆ 1 Tb balsamic vinegar ◆ 1 2-lb butternut squash seeded and quartered (skin left on) ◆ 1 tsp Dijon mustard ◆ Salt and ground white pepper ◆ 1 Tb liquid sweetener

Mushrooms, Broiled

Use large caps for broiling. Spray with zero-calorie butter spray. Place on broiler rack, cap side up, about 4 inches from the broiling unit. Broil 2 to 2 1/2 minutes, then turn them over. Add a dash of salt, pepper, and/or Tabasco sauce into each cap. Cook another 2 1/2 minutes. Serving ideas: Top with allowable portion of butter, parsley, dill, and/or bacon.

Ingredients

1 pound mushrooms ◆ zero-calorie butter spray ◆ salt ◆ pepper ◆ Tabasco sauce

Mushrooms, Grilled Portabello

Remove stems of mushrooms, and wipe them with a damp cloth. Preheat the broiler or grill. Mix vinegar, herbs, and garlic in a bowl. Spray mushrooms with zero-calorie butter spray. Brush mushrooms with the vinegar mixture. Grill or broil the mushrooms 3-5 minutes per side, or until soft and brown. Measure 1 cup and serve.

Ingredients

6 medium portabello mushrooms ◆ 1 teaspoon fresh rosemary or 1/2 teaspoon dried rosemary ◆ 3 tablespoons balsamic vinegar ◆ 1 teaspoon fresh thyme or 1/2 teaspoon dried thyme ◆ 2 cloves garlic thinly sliced ◆ salt and pepper

Mushrooms, Sauteed

Wash well and dry. Do not peel. Trim stems, if desired.Spray skillet with zero-calorie butter spray. Turn heat to medium. When butter spray begins to bubble, add mushrooms. Saute over medium heat 6 to 8 minutes. Shake the pan several times to reduce heat slightly. Measure 1 cup and serve. Serving ideas: Top with allowable portion of butter, parsley, dill, and/or bacon.

Ingredients

1 pound mushrooms quartered, whole, or sliced
◆ zero-calorie butter spray ◆ salt ◆ pepper

Mushrooms, Sauteed

Wash well and dry. Do not peel. Trim stems, if desired.Spray skillet with zero-calorie butter spray. Turn heat to medium. When butter spray begins to bubble, add mushrooms. Saute over medium heat 6 to 8 minutes. Shake the pan several times to reduce heat slightly. Measure 1 cup and serve. Serving ideas: Top with allowable portion of butter, parsley, dill, and/or bacon.

Ingredients

1 pound mushrooms quartered, whole, or sliced
◆ zero-calorie butter spray ◆ salt ◆ pepper

Mushrooms, Steamed

Wash well and dry. Do not peel. Trim stems, if desired. Pour 1/4 inch water in a covered heavy saucepan and bring to a gentle boil with lemon juice and salt. Add the mushrooms, cover, and steam about 5 minutes, shaking the pan occasionally, so mushrooms do not stick to the bottom.

Ingredients

1 pound mushrooms ◆ 1 tablespoon lemon juice ◆ 1 teaspoon salt

New World Pumpkin

Bring water to a boil, cover, and simmer over medium heat until the water has evaporated, stirring occasionally to prevent sticking. Measure and serve.

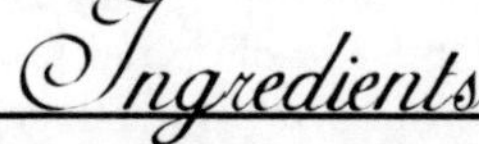

◆ 1 large onion, chopped
◆ 6 assorted fresh mild green chilies seeded and chopped
◆ 2 cloves garlic chopped ◆ 1 lb fresh pumpkin or winter squash peeled and cubed ◆ 1 small can chopped tomatoes (or 2 fresh tomatoes chopped) ◆ salt

Okra, Steamed

Wash the okra well and cut off the stems. If the pods are young, leave whole. If older, cut in slices. Steam-cook in a small amount of boiling salted water about 10 minutes, or till just tender. Overcooking tends to give it a disagreeable texture. Measure 1 cup and serve. Serving ideas: Top with allowable portion of butter or olive oil.

Ingredients

1 pound small okra ◆ salt

Okra, Stir-Fried

Cut the both ends off each okra, and then cut them in two halves lengthwise. Spray sauce pan with zero-calorie butter spray. Add chopped garlic and ginger and fry for 5 minutes. Stir in okra. Sprinkle salt, and add chopped jalapeno (optional). Cook for 8-10 minutes, but stir after every 1-2 minute till okra is tender. Sprinkle freshly ground pepper on top. Measure 1 cup and serve. Variation: Add 1 sliced, medium onion, to pan with okra, and measure 1/2 cup serving.

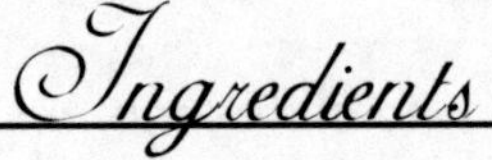

1 pound okra ◆ 4 - 5 cloves garlic peeled and chopped ◆ 1 tablespoon ginger, peeled and chopped finely ◆ salt ◆ jalapeno ◆ optional

Olive Oil Garlic Broccoli

Sprinkle Garlic Powder on Raw Broccoli. Steam Broccoli. Toss with 1 tablespoons Olive Oil. Cover and continue to steam covered on its own about 5 minutes. Measure and serve.

Ingredients

16 oz Broccoli or 2 cups ◆ 1 Tbs Olive Oil
◆ Dash Garlic Powder

Onion Squash à la Sophie's Choice

Place the cubes of squash into a large saucepan with the onion, garlic, 1 Tb butter, and thyme. Cover and sweat over low heat for 10 minutes, stirring occasionally. Add the tomatoes, salt, pepper, and nutmeg. Stir thoroughly and cook, covered, over low heat until squash is very tender. Discard thyme stalk. Grind coriander, cumin, and peppercorns coarsely. Melt the remaining 1 Tb butter in a small bowl (or pan, if you are not equipped with a microwave) and add the crushed spices, mustard seeds, and cinnamon. Mix into squash just before serving.

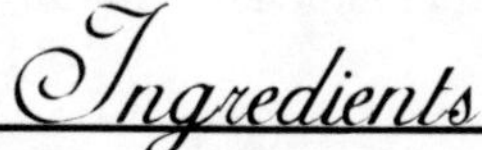

2 lb peeled and seeded winter squash cut into cubes
◆ 1 onion chopped ◆ 2 cloves of garlic chopped
◆ 1 Tb butter ◆ 1 can diced tomatoes ◆ 1 sprig fresh thyme or 1 tsp dried thyme/salt/pepper/nutmeg ◆ 1/2 tsp coriander seeds ◆ 1/2 tsp cumin seeds ◆ 1/2 tsp black peppercorns
◆ 1 tsp white mustard seeds ◆ 2 in piece cinnamon stick broken up

Onion Squash alla Milanese

An hour or two before you plan to start preparing your meal, cut the squash in two, remove seeds, and bake face-down on a foil-lined tray at 400° F until the squash is easily pierced by a fork (approximately 40 minutes). Remove from oven and set aside until cool enough to handle. Scoop out of the shell and mash to an even consistency. (Note: you can skip this stage by using frozen or canned squash. The remainder of the preparation will be the same.) Heat 1 1/2 tsp. of the butter in a large, deep skillet and sauté onions and garlic until very soft. Add the remaining 11/2 tsp butter, squash, sage, bay leaf, basil, and considerable quantities of salt and pepper. (Squash absorbs spices like a sponge.) Stir to mix well and let cook 2 minutes. Add the vinegar and stir thoroughly. Lower heat and allow to cook for 15 to 20 minutes more, stirring occasionally.

Ingredients

1 large onion squash ◆ 1 large red onion finely chopped ◆ 3 cloves garlic peeled and chopped ◆ 2 whole sage leaves or 2 tsp rubbed sage ◆ 1 bay leaf ◆ 3 Tb white vinegar, small handful of fresh basil leaves torn into small pieces ◆ salt and pepper ◆ 1 Tb butter

Onions, Boiled

Drop trimmed and peeled onions into boiling salted water. Cook small ones for 15 minutes, large ones for 30 minutes. They should be pierceable with a fork, yet firm. Measure 1/2 cup and serve. Serving ideas: Top with allowable portion of butter, pepper, salt, nutmeg, and mace. Top with portion of cheddar or Gruyere cheese. Top with tomato sauce.

Ingredients

3 onions ◆ salt

Onions, Broiled

Cut onions into thick slices. Spray grilling pan with zero-calorie butter spray. Arrange onion slices on grilling pan. Spray onion slices with zero-calorie butter spray. Top with salt. Broil about 4 inches from heat unit. When they are brown, turn them carefully, with spatulas. Spray and salt other side. Return to broiler to brown second side. Measure 1/2 cup and serve.

Ingredients

onions ◆ zero-calorie butter spray

Onions, Steamed

Trim, peel, and slice onions. Spray heavy saucepan with zero-calorie butter spray. Add sliced onions, salt, nutmeg or mace, and cover tightly. Steam over low heat approximately 10 minutes. Shake the pan gently a few times during the cooking. Measure 1/2 cup and serve.

Ingredients

4 - 8 onions ◆ zero-calorie butter spray ◆ 1 teaspoon salt ◆ dash of nutmeg or mace

Orange Squash Crunch

Take it out of the cardboard. Spray w/butter flavored PAM and put on a dish. Sprinkle w/cinnamon and nuke forever until crunchy. Serve with drizzled sesame oil, butter or Loriva peanut oil and add soy nuts or cheese too!

Ingredients

1 Box Orange Frozen Squash

Pennsylvania Dutch Fried Cabbage

Add cabbage to olive oil in frying pan. Cook on high for 5 minutes to lightly browned. Turn heat down. Cover cabbage and cook, tossing lightly occasionally, for about 20 minutes.

Ingredients

2-3 cups Green Cabbage ◆ 1 tablespoons Olive Oil or other oil

Peppers, Sautéed

Clean, seed, and cut peppers in julienne strips or in rounds. Heat allowable portion of olive oil in skillet over low heat. Add garlic, thinly sliced. Let it melt in the oil about 4 minutes. Add the peppers and cover. Let them steam in the oil, shaking the pan occasionally, till just soft - about 15 to 20 minutes. Add the salt. Serving ideas: Serve with beef, chicken, or pork.

Ingredients

3 green, red, or yellow bell peppers◆ 1 1/2 tsp olive oil ◆ 1/2 clove of garlic◆ salt

Pizza

Bake crust at 550 for about 10 minutes. Add toppings and bake for 5 more minutes, until cheese is cooked to your liking.

Ingredients

1 1/4 oz. wheat germ ◆ 1/2 oz soy flour ◆ garlic powder ◆ basil ◆ oregano ◆ salt ◆ pepper ◆ seltzer ◆ 1 or 2 tsp olive oil ◆ 5 oz. pasta sauce ◆ 5 oz. Mushrooms (or other cooked vegetables) ◆ 1.5 oz. fake sausage ◆ 1 oz. cheese

Portuguese Peppers

Heat the oil and butter in a skillet over medium heat. Add the peppers, onions, garlic, salt, and pepper. Cook about 3 minutes or until crisp and tender. Add tomato sauce and saffron. Cover and simmer 15 minutes.

Ingredients

1 tablespoon olive oil ◆ 1 tablespoon butter ◆ 3 cups cored and seeded red, green, and yellow peppers, cut into thin strips ◆ 1 medium onion, finely chopped ◆ 1 tablespoon finely chopped fresh garlic ◆ salt and freshly-ground pepper ◆ 1/2 cup tomato sauce ◆ 1/4 teaspoon saffron or 1/2 teaspoon turmeric

Potato Pancakes

First cook squash 10 minutes or so in microwave. Measure. Fry with spices. And 1 egg with olive oil and peanut oil Cover cook like an omelet.

Ingredients

Spaghetti Squash ◆ 1 egg ◆ 1 tsp Olive Oil or Peanut Oil

Pumpkin as a Heated Vegetable

Combine ingredients. Heat in pan.

Ingredients

1/2 or 4 ozs pumpkin ◆ 1 tsp butter

Pumpkin Cream Puree

Mix all ingredients in one bowl. Simmer on stove, or cook in microwave for several minutes. Great for Thanksgiving!

Ingredients

1/2 cup pumpkin ◆ 1 cup milk ◆ 1/2 teaspoon cinnamon ◆ 1/4 teaspoon ginger ◆ 1/4 teaspoon salt ◆ dash of clove ◆ sweetener

Pumpkin Loaf

Preheat oven to 400°F. Beat the egg, water, spices, and salt together in a large bowl with a whisk. Add ground texturized soy protein and beat until smooth. Fold in pumpkin with a large spatula. Spray mini-loaf pan heavily with Pam. Pour the pumpkin mixture into the pan and bake for 30-40 minutes. When serving, slice lengthwise and reheat, if desired. Top with sweetener, cinnamon and zero calorie butter spray. Great for traveling!

Ingredients

1 egg ◆ 2 ounces ground texturized soy protein ◆ 1/2 cup pumpkin ◆ 1/4 cup water ◆ 1 teaspoon each: cinnamon, nutmeg, ginger, allspice ◆ 1 teaspoon salt ◆ zero calorie butter spray ◆ sweetener

Pumpkin Mock Pie w/o crust

Combine ingredients. Heat or chill.

Ingredients

1/2 c or 4 ozs pumpkin ◆ sweetener ◆ nutmeg ◆ cinnamon

Pumpkin Muffin

Combine ingredients. Microwave for 2 minutes on high.

Ingredients

1/8 cup wheat germ ◆ 1 oz pure pumpkin ◆ 2 packets Equal
◆ splash of cinnamon
◆ 1/2 cap of walnut flavor (sugar-free, alcohol free, oil free)
◆ 1/2 cap of maple flavor (sugar-free, alcohol free, oil free)

Pumpkin Pie

Mix together, pour into abstinent sprayed custard cup and bake at 350 degrees for 30 to 35 minutes.

Ingredients

1/8 cup wheat germ ◆ 1 oz pure pumpkin ◆ 2 packets Equal
◆ splash of cinnamon
◆ 1/2 cap of walnut flavor (sugar-free, alcohol free, oil free)
◆ 1/2 cap of maple flavor (sugar-free, alcohol free, oil free)

Pumpkin Refritos

Place the ancho chile in a small saucepan and cover with water. Bring to a boil. Reduce heat and simmer until chile is soft, about 10 minutes. Remove the chile from the liquid. When it is cool enough to handle, stem the chile, split it open, and scrape out the seeds. Place the pumpkin in a food processor and add the chile, cumin, salt, and cayenne pepper. Process until smooth, stopping to scrape down the sides of the bowl. Transfer to an oven-proof dish and bake at 350° until the top is crusty.

Ingredients

1 dried ancho chile ◆ 1-2 cans pumpkin ◆ 1/4 teaspoon ground cumin ◆ 1 teaspoon salt, plus more to taste ◆ scant pinch cayenne pepper

Pumpkin Souffle-Pudding

Blend ingredients. Add spices and sweetener to taste.

Ingredients

1/2 c pumpkin or 4 ozs pumpkin ◆ 1 c yogurt

Pumpkin With Wheat Germ

In a safe microwave container weight and measure the pumpkin/squash. Then add wheat germ, add pinch of salt, cinnamon, vanilla flavoring (sometimes I'll buy almond flavoring- not too often its expensive), equal, add seltzer/cream soda. Use enough soda/seltzer etc. to cover the veggies for moisture, let it sit for 30 seconds to a minute. The wheat germ will soak up and expand from the liquids. Then put in the microwave for 2-4 minutes depending on your microwave. Then I usually use 1 tablespoon butter on top. Let it cool for a few minutes.

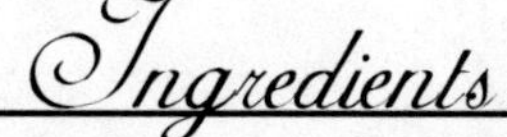

2oz Pumpkin or Squash ◆ 1 tbs Wheat Germ
◆ Diet Cream soda or seltzer, (you can also use water too I just add extra vanilla flavoring when I use water)

Pumpkin Yogurt Delight

Bring pumpkin to a boil in the microwave. Add allowable portion of butter, cinnamon, and sweetener; mix well. Add yogurt, stir thoroughly, and freeze for 2 hours. Makes 1/2 protein and 1 cooked vegetable.

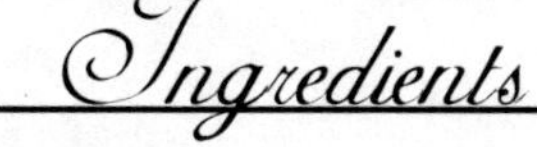

1/2 cup yogurt ◆ 1/2 cup pumpkin
◆ 1/2 teaspoon cinnamon ◆ sweetener

Pumpkin Yummy

Stir ingredients together. Microwave or bake until the cheese melts.

Ingredients

4 oz canned pumpkin W/O sugar ◆ cinnamon and cloves (LITTLE BIT) ◆ 1 egg ◆ 1/8 cup wheat germ ◆ 1 oz soy Cheddar cheese ◆ 1 oz soy nuts

Pumpkin, Baked

Cut the Pumpkin in half. Remove the seeds. Bake at 350 F, covered in a small amount of water until tender. Scoop the pulp out. Measure 1/2 cup and serve. Serving ideas: Serve hot with allowable portion of butter, pumpkin pie spice, and sweetener. Serve cold stirred into yogurt for pudding!

Ingredients

1 pumpkin

Pumpkin-Yogurt Unbaked Soufflé

Blend. Eat with a spoon.

Ingredients

1/2 cup uncooked canned "100% pure Pumpkin" ◆ 1 cup Plain Yogurt ◆ Nutmeg and Cinnamon to taste

Rajas Con Jitomate

Remove the seeds and veins from the chiles and cut them into strips about 1 1/2 inches long and 1/2 inch wide. (You may want to substitute anaheim chiles for poblanos--they are milder.) Heat the oil and fry the onions gently, without browning them, until they are soft. Add the chile strips, tomatoes and salt to the onions in the pan. Cook uncovered over a fairly high flame until the vegetables are well seasoned and the liquid has evaporated.

Ingredients

8 chiles poblano chiles roasted and peeled ◆ 1 Tb peanut oil ◆ 1 1/2 medium onions thinly sliced ◆ 1 tsp salt ◆ 2 cans chopped tomatoes drained

Ratatouille

Coat skillet with butter-type spray (check with sponsor) Cook onions & garlic in the vinegar and water, then add green peppers, cook a bit, add zucchini, cook a bit more, then add rest of ingredients. Add water and/or vinegar as necessary to keep it from burning.

Ingredients

1 large Eggplant ◆ peeled and cubed ◆ 1 large Zucchini sliced and peeled ◆ Tomato Paste to taste ◆ Green Peppers, cored and de-seeded ◆ Onions, peeled and sliced into rounds then into quarters or use Onion Seasoning ◆ Fresh Garlic, chopped or just peeled ◆ Vinegar ◆ Water as needed to keep mixture from burning ◆ Salt & Pepper to taste ◆ Oregano ◆ Basil ◆ Bay Leaf

Red Bell Peppers

Cut peppers in one-half lengthwise. Take out core and seeds. Place peppers cut-side up in a jellyroll pan or on a cookie sheet. (I use parchment paper underneath.) Measure allotted amount per Greysheet portion for meal.

Ingredients

Red Bell Peppers or Yellow or Orange Sweet Peppers

Roasted Cauliflower

Break cauliflower into florets. Toss in olive oil to coat lightly. Spread in baking pan. Add salt and pepper to taste. Bake at 375 degrees for 20 minutes. Turn and bake another 10 minutes or until golden.

Ingredients

1 head cauliflower ◆ freshly ground sea salt ◆ freshly ground pepper

Roasted Mixed Vegetables

I take a whole cauliflower and whole bunch of broccoli. Clean and wash well. Drain. Place in a large pan. Add about 1 tablespoon of oil. Season to taste. I like using SEASON-ALL. It is a seasoned salt. Toss together. Roast this at the same time you are roasting chicken. I stir it about once every 1/2 hour. I leave it in the oven for about 2 hours. It comes out cooked but not mushy.

Ingredients

1 head cauliflower ◆ 1 Tb. olive oil ◆ freshly ground sea salt ◆ freshly ground pepper

Roasted Peppers

Halve and core peppers and place skin-side-up on a baking sheet. Roast under broiler until skins turn black and peppers are soft. Place in paper bag and allow to cool; close top of bag and shake until skins are loose. Finish removing skins, slice peppers into strips, and combine with lemon juice, salt, and pepper. Weigh and measure and serve..

Ingredients

2 Red Bell Peppers ◆ 2 Gold Bell Peppers ◆ 2 Green Bell Peppers ◆ 2 tablespoons Lemon juice ◆ Salt and Pepper

Roasted Vegetables

Slice rutabaga thin and lay them out on aluminum foil on a pan. I spray the pan first, then lay the slices, cover them with salt, pepper, dill, or any other seasoning that appeals (cinnamon isn't bad -- along with some Indian spices), try oregano and thyme, then spray again!!! Roast in oven for 20 minutes or thereabouts -- you can tell they are done if the edges start to look burnt!

Ingredients

Butter flavor spay ◆ ◆ zero-calorie butter spray ◆ Seasonings

Roasted Vegetables Terrine

Slice rutabaga thin and lay them out on aluminum foil on a pan. I spray the pan first, then lay the slices, cover them with salt, pepper, dill, or any other seasoning that appeals (cinnamon isn't bad -- along with some Indian spices), try oregano and thyme, then spray again!!! Once all of the veggies are layered, cover with saran wrap and place in the refrigerator overnight (even better with something on top to weigh it down). To serve, cut, as you would pie.

Ingredients

Eggplants cut into circles ◆ Zucchini cut into strips ◆ Red pepper whole (place in plastic bag after cooked until cooled for easy peeling) any other vegetable you like ◆ 1 bag of fresh spinach ◆ crushed garlic ◆ seasonings to taste

Roasted Vidalia Onions

Peel the onions and core with a knife or apple corer. Try not to go all the way through, so that you've made sort of a well. (You may need to use a grapefruit spoon to achieve this.) Divide the butter in half and put one part in the well of each onion. Lightly salt & pepper each onion and wrap in aluminum foil. Place on a moderately hot spot of a grill for 45 minutes to an hour. A knife should go through it like butter. Whatever you do, it'll be good, but perfection is almost black on the bottom where the onion sugars have almost burned & very tender on the inside. This is intended to make 1 8-oz serving.

Ingredients

2 medium Vidalia onions ◆ 1 Tb Butter ◆ Salt and Pepper

Rutabaga

Peel raw rutabaga with peeler. Carefully poke holes in rutabaga, by stabbing with a fork. Wrap with plastic wrap or moist paper towel. Microwave for 5-7 minutes. Remove from microwave. Let cool for 10 minutes. Leave plastic wrap on to steam while cooling. Remove wrap. Dice rutabaga into small cubes. Measure 1/2 cup and serve.

Ingredients

1 fresh rutabaga

Rutabaga - Cleaning & Preparation

Put the waxy colored globe on a cutting board. Take the strong knife and at the side of the globe, cut a 1/2 inch round slice (like you were cutting a cucumber slice). Continue cutting slices. Then peel the wax outer coat from around each slice and discard. Place the yellow round peeled slices on your cutting board. Cut them crosswise in 1/2 to 3/4 inch strips. Then cut these strips crosswise to make small cubes. To cook, microwave the cubes for 6 minutes on high or boil the cubes until tender. Mash the cubes and add butter or oil. Microwave or stovetop.

Ingredients

rutabaga ◆ 1 Tb butter or oil

Rutabaga, Boiled

Peel rutabaga. Cut into dice or slices. Cook in boiling, salted water, to cover, over medium heat until they are just tender. Drain well. Mash with masher, mixer or fork, if desired. Measure 1/2 cup and serve with allowable portion of butter. Also known as swedes or yellow turnips. Measure 1/2 cup serving.

Ingredients

1 large rutabaga ◆ salt ◆ pepper ◆ allowable portion of butter

Rutabaga, Microwaved

Peel raw rutabaga with peeler. Carefully poke holes in rutabaga, by stabbing with a fork. Wrap with plastic wrap or moist paper towel. Microwave for 5-7 minutes. Remove from microwave. Let cool for 10 minutes. Leave plastic wrap on to steam while cooling. Remove wrap. Dice rutabaga into small cubes. Measure 1/2 cup and serve. These are great tater substitutes! Measure 1/2 cup serving.

Ingredients

1 large rutabaga

Saffron Shallots

Soak the saffron threads in the vinegar and sweetener for at least 20 minutes. Heat the olive oil in a heavy-bottomed saucepan and add the shallots, garlic, chili, and saffron liquid, including saffron threads. (Note: this works with Turkish ground saffron as well.) Soak the saffron threads in the vinegar and sweetener for at least 20 minutes. Heat the olive oil in a heavy-bottomed saucepan and add the shallots, garlic, chili, and saffron liquid, including saffron threads. (Note: this works with Turkish ground saffron as well.)

Ingredients

2 lbs small whole shallots peeled and trimmed ◆ 3 cloves garlic chopped ◆ 1 small red chili finely chopped small pinch saffron threads ◆ 1 tsp liquid sweetener ◆ 2 Tb white vinegar ◆ 1 Tb olive oil ◆ salt and pepper

Salad, Taco Style

Measure out taco-style salad vegetables, such as lettuce, tomato, carrots, etc. Stir cooked ground beef or soy in with cooked onions and tomato sauce. Top salad with cooked meat and onions. Add allowable portion of ranch dressing on top.

Ingredients

2 cups salad ◆ 4 ounces cooked ground beef or 4 ounces cooked ground soy, such as Gimme Lean ◆ 1/2 cup sauteed onions ◆ 2 ounces tomato sauce, taco spices or abstinent seasoned salt, ranch dressing

Samba Squash

Pierce the squash several times with a knife, place on a heatproof dish, and microwave on high until soft, turning frequently. (About 10-15 minutes.) Remove from microwave, slice open to reveal seeds, and allow to cool for a few minutes. While the squash is nuking, boil the carrots on the stovetop until extremely soft. When they are finished, drain and transfer to a large mixing bowl. Scoop the flesh out of the squash (first removing seeds) and add to the bowl. Add the butter and ginger. Mash thoroughly. (I personally recommend using a hand-mixer unless you have a lot of frustrations to get out.) Season generously with salt and pepper. Serve hot.

Ingredients

2 sweet dumpling squash ◆ 1/8 tsp ground ginger ◆ 6 medium carrots, cut into 1-inch chunks ◆ salt and black pepper ◆ 3 tsp.sweet butter

Sauerkraut and Bacon, Fried

Measure out taco-style salad vegetables, such as lettuce, tomato, carrots, etc. Stir cooked ground beef or soy in with cooked onions and tomato sauce. Top salad with cooked meat and onions. Add allowable portion of ranch dressing on top.

Ingredients

4 ounces bacon or cut up frankfurters ◆ 8 ounces sauerkraut drained ◆ salt and pepper, margarine

Sauteed Spinach

Weigh 8 ozs spinach, fresh, washed and clean. Put 1 tbs olive oil in hot pan. Saute 3 garlic cloves and fresh spinach quickly on high heat. Cover and steam for 1 minute.Also works with kale, collard greens, mustard greens, turnip greens. Garlic and olice oil are the secret.

Ingredients

Fresh spinach ◆ 1 tablespoon olive oil ◆ 3 pressed garlic cloves

Sautéed Squash in Herb Sauce

Thinly slice onion, peel and dice squash. Sauté sliced onion in olive oil. Add pepper, celery seed, oregano, and cumin; stir. Add squash and stir to mix. Add water and vinegar and cook over medium heat, stirring constantly, until squash is very tender.

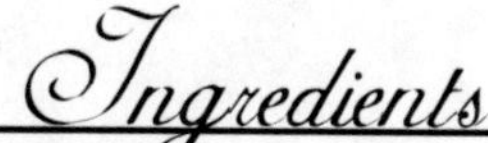

1 medium onion thinly sliced ◆ 1 Tb olive oil ◆ 1/4 tsp ground pepper ◆ 1/4 tsp celery seed ◆ 1/4 tsp oregano ◆ dash of cumin ◆ 1 large squash peeled and diced ◆ 1/2 cup water ◆ 2 Tb white vinegar

Savory Pumpkin Stew

Sauté onion and garlic in oil until transparent, about 4 minutes. Add pumpkin and turnips and cook, stirring occasionally, for 5 minutes. Add water, 1 cup at a time, until there is enough liquid in the pot to simmer the vegetables. Stir in mustard, cinnamon and vinegar. Simmer uncovered, stirring occasionally, over medium-low heat for 30 minutes or until water has nearly evaporated and vegetables are tender. (If water evaporates too soon, add a bit more.) Add green beans and cook 5 minutes more. Season to taste with salt and pepper. This works with rutabagas substituted for the pumpkin.

Ingredients

1 Onion diced ◆ 1 medium Pumpkin peeled seeded and cut into cubes ◆ 2 Turnips peeled and chopped ◆ 1 small package frozen cut Green Beans ◆ 3 cloves Garlic minced ◆ 1 tablespoon Apple Cider Vinegar ◆ 2 tablespoons Mustard ◆ 1 teaspoon ground Cinnamon ◆ Salt and Pepper ◆ 1 tablespoon Vegetable Oil

Spanakopita

Mix ingredients together.. Bake in sprayed pyrex dish, 350 degrees, 30-40 minutes.

Ingredients

8 oz. spinach ◆ cooked and drained ◆ dried onion flakes ◆ fresh chopped dill ◆ one egg ◆ one oz. Crumbled feta cheese

Shoko Spinach

Reserve 1/2 cup of juice from the canned tomatoes, and discard the rest of the juice. Combine the chile, onions, and green bell pepper in a food processor, and process until the vegetables are minced but not pureed. Heat the oil in a large heavy pot, and sauté the vegetables for 5 minutes over high heat. Add the reserved tomato juice, water, sweetener, salt, cayenne, and ginger. Add the spinach to the pot a little at a time. (It will wilt, shrink, and leave you room to add more.) Cook over medium heat for 30 minutes, until the water is gone and the spinach is cooked.

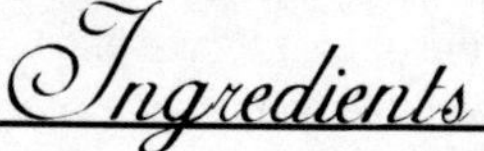

1 small can chopped tomatoes drained ◆ 1 fresh hot chili seeded and chopped ◆ 4 medium onions coarsely chopped ◆ 1 green bell pepper seeded and chopped ◆ 1 tablespoon vegetable oil ◆ 1/4 teaspoon liquid sweetener ◆ 1/2 teaspoon salt ◆ 1 teaspoon cayenne pepper ◆ 1 1/2 teaspoon grated fresh ginger ◆ 2 lbs fresh spinach washed and coarsely shredded

Spaghetti Squash alla Marinara

Combine capers, basil, garlic, oil, and tomato sauce in saucepan. Allow to stand 30 minutes. Prepare spaghetti squash as in above recipe. While squash is cooking, simmer sauce over low heat until oil has absorbed sauce. Add cooked squash to sauce and mix thoroughly. Weigh as regular 8 oz. vegetable.

Ingredients

1 spaghetti squash ◆ small can tomato sauce or crushed tomatoes ◆ 1 tablespoon capers ◆ 4 or 5 leaves fresh basil ◆ 4 or 5 cloves garlic pressed ◆ 1 tablespoon olive oil

Sicilian Sweet and Sour Pumpkin

Preheat the oven to 375°. Cut the pumpkin in half and remove the seeds. Place cut side down on a baking sheet and bake about 45 minutes or until tender but not mushy. The pumpkin flesh should be firm enough to peel and cut into 1/2-inch cubes or slices. Sprinkle with salt and pepper. While pumpkin is baking, bring 1 cup water to a boil in a small, deep saucepan. Add onions and butter and cook, uncovered, over moderate heat until tender. When most of the liquid has evaporated, sprinkle the onions with sweetener and cook until the onions begin to caramelize. Add the vinegar and 1 cup water. Continue to cook until deep golden brown but not burned. Add water if the mixture seems dry; the onions should end up in a sweet and sour syrup. Toss the pumpkin cubes with the onions and stir well to coat. Sprinkle with coarsely chopped mint.

Ingredients

2 lb Pumpkin or butternut squash ◆ 3 onions, finely sliced ◆ 1 tablespoons butter ◆ 1 tablespoon sweetener ◆ 3 tablespoons balsamic vinegar ◆ Salt and pepper ◆ 1/2 cup fresh mint chopped

Spanakopita (Spinach)

Mix together and bake in sprayed Pyrex dish 350 degrees, 30-40 minutes.

Ingredients

8 oz. spinach, cooked and drained ◆ dried onion flakes ◆ fresh chopped dill ◆ 1 egg ◆ 1 oz. Feta cheese-crumbled

Sautéed Squash in Herb Sauce

Mix everything in a food processor or blender until smooth. When weighing the tomatoes and mushrooms, you may wish to include some of the juices from the tomatoes in your measurement to help the consistency of the dip. Pour the processed or blended mixture into a microwaveable container and heat on high for about 3 minutes (more if your microwave is lower wattage). You can use that time to clean and ready your raw veggies. *Can be fresh (raw) but you should increase your cooking time accordingly.

Ingredients

3 ounces canned soy beans* ◆ 1 ounce grated or shredded soy cheese ◆ 8 ounces canned chopped tomatoes with green chiles (sometimes sold by the brand name RoTel) and drained canned mushrooms* ◆ 1/4 to 1/2 teaspoon hot red pepper flakes ◆ 1/2 teaspoon garlic powder ◆ 1 teaspoon onion powder ◆ 1/2 teaspoon ground celery seed (celery powder) ◆ 1/2 teaspoon salt (or to taste) ◆ Raw veggies from Lunch Finger Salad or Dinner Salad

Spicy Green Peppers

Remove stem and seeds from green peppers. Cut into long slices. Heat oil in a pan and fry pepper slices until light brown. Remove from pan and add mustard seeds. When mustard seeds begin to pop, add onions; cook 4-5 minutes over medium heat. Add cumin, salt, and cayenne; stir and cook for a few minutes. Return peppers to pot, and 1/2 cup water, and bring to a boil. Simmer 3-4 minutes and serve hot.

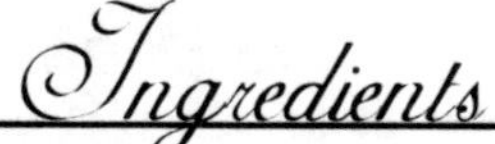

6 medium sized green peppers ◆ 2 medium onions ◆ finely chopped ◆ 1 tsp mustard seeds ◆ 1 Tb ground cumin ◆ 1/2 tsp cayenne ◆ 3 Tb lemon juice ◆ salt to taste ◆ 1 Tb vegetable oil

Soy Pizza

Weigh soy flour. Add enough water to soy flour to make a ball. Spray hands liberally with zero-calorie butter spray. Shape soy flour into ball, and then spread out as thin as possible. Pan fry in pan liberally coated in zero-calorie butter spray. Microwave pepperoni in paper towels. Saute mushrooms in zero-calorie butter spray and garlic. Weigh and measure cooked pepperoni and mushrooms. Layer all on cooked soy flour and serve. Serving Variations: Use 1 oz. soy cheese by reducing soy flour and pepperoni to 1 1/2 oz. each. Use 3/4 cup mushrooms and 1/4 cup chopped tomatoes with green chiles (RoTel). Use 1 cup artichoke hearts and 1 oz. roquefort cheese instead of mushrooms and pepperoni. Season soy flour with abstinent spices or allowable portion of juice from canned tomatoes or jalapeno peppers.

Ingredients

2 ounces soy flour or finely ground texturized soy protein ◆ 2 ounces pepperoni ◆ 1 cup mushrooms ◆ zero-calorie butter spray, garlic

Spinach

Frozen spinach cooked in the microwave. Measure 8oz. Add salt pepper, garlic powder, paprika. Then 2 tablespoons of mayo. Mix. Eat. Its like a spinach dip. Make sure you flavor it well. You may have to add an extra dash of salt. (you could even add w/m Parmesan or Romano cheese but you would have to take from you allotted proteins)

Ingredients

Frozen Spinach ◆ Salt ◆ Pepper ◆ Garlic Powder ◆ Paprika ◆ 1 tablespoons Mayo

Soy Pizza, Large Crust

Preheat oven to 550° F or as hot as it will go. Heat the pizza stone or baking sheet inside the oven. Mix texturized soy protein, garlic powder, salt, oil, and cold water to form a firm ball of dough (use a fork). Add the water a little at a time to avoid making an unusable mess. Roll between sheets of non-stick baking paper until you have a flat pizza about 1/2 inch thick. Place dough on the preheated pizza stone or pizza pan. Bake for 5 minutes, until dry and somewhat golden. Remove from oven, spread the vegetables and tomato sauce, and bake for another 8 minutes.

Ingredients

4 ounces finely ground texturized soy protein ◆ 1 teaspoon garlic powder ◆ salt ◆ 1 tablespoon sesame oil (fat from salad) or 2 teaspoon zero calorie butter spray, approx ◆ 1/4 cup water ◆ 1 cup cooked vegetables, such as zucchini, mushrooms, tomatoes with Italian seasonings ◆ 2 ounces tomato sauce

Soy Pizza, Small Crust

Preheat oven to 425° F. Brush the oil over a baking sheet or pizza pan. Mix texturized soy protein, salt, and about 2 Tbl. water in a bowl, and combine to form dough. Roll between sheets of non-stick baking paper until you have a flat crust, or spread with your fingers onto a baking sheet. Spread the tomato sauce on top with a brush or spatula. Sprinkle the pepperoni and soy cheese on top. Bake for 10-15 minutes.

Ingredients

2 ounces finely ground texturized soy protein ◆ 1 ounce pepperoni ◆ 1 ounce grated mozzarella soy cheese ◆ 1 teaspoon salt, ◆ 2 ounces tomato paste/sauce mixed with Italian seasoning (or diet catsup may be substituted)

Spinach and Portabello Mushrooms, Sauteed

Spray skillet or sauté pan with zero-calorie butter spray. Over medium heat, sauté vegetables and spices until mushrooms are tender, and spinach is heated through. Measure 1 cup and serve. Variation: Top with grated parmesan cheese as measured portion of protein.

Ingredients

2 large portabello mushrooms sliced ◆ 1 10-ounce package frozen chopped spinach, thawed and drained ◆ 1/4 teaspoon dried basil ◆ 1/4 teaspoon salt ◆ 1/4 teaspoon black pepper ◆ 1 clove garlic ◆ chopped ◆ zero-calorie butter spray

Spinach Casserole

Mix all together and microwave to heat.

Ingredients

4 oz. cottage cheese ◆ 8 oz. frozen spinach (thawed) or 4 oz. spinach and 1 tablespoon wheat germ ◆ 1 tablespoon butter ◆ 1/2 teaspoon salt ◆ 1 teaspoon nutmeg

Spinach Quiche

Beat egg in a straight-sided plastic container. Add wheat germ, salt, pepper, and spices of your choice. Add spinach and cheese. Top with allowable portion of butter. Microwave about 4 minutes. Makes a good travel food, and tastes good hot or cold!

Ingredients

1 egg ◆ 1 ounce feta cheese ◆ 1 tablespoon wheat germ ◆ 1/2 cup cooked spinach ◆ salt ◆ pepper ◆ spices ◆ butter

Spinach or Chard, Sauteed with Garlic

Trim and clean the spinach, cut into palm size pieces. In a large pan, spray zero-calorie butter spray. Cook the garlic and red pepper in the pan over medium heat, until the garlic is golden. Add the spinach and salt to taste. Stir well. Cover the pot and cook until spinach is tender, just a few minutes. Measure 1 cup. Serve hot or at room temperature.

Ingredients

1 bunch fresh spinach or chard (any greens)
◆ 3 cloves garlic, thinly sliced ◆ 1 pinch crushed red pepper flakes
◆ salt ◆ zero-calorie butter spray (olive flavor is good)

Spinach Stroganoff

Cut Tempeh into chunks, slices, whatever. Mix with cooked onions and oil, heat in non-stick pan. Prepare Tofu Sour Cream by combining all ingredients in blender adding enough water and blending till smooth. Combine Tempeh mixture with Tofu Sour Cream mixture. Add spinach and cook until warm.

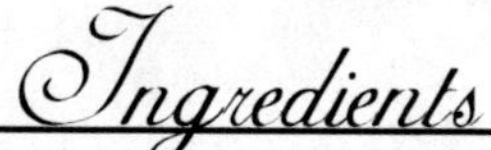

2 oz. Tempeh ◆ 1 teaspoon olive oil
◆ ¼ cup onion (cooked in microwave) ◆ ½ cup cooked spinach.
◆ 2 oz. firm tofu ◆ ½ teaspoon lemon concentrate
◆ 2 teaspoons soy sauce ◆ 1 teaspoon olive oil
◆ salt to taste ◆ water for blending

Spinach, Steamed

Wash spinach well. Warm water removes dirt more easily. Discard heavier stems. Put washed spinach in a large heavy saucepan and cover. Add no water. Steam it until it is just wilted thoroughly - about 5 to 8 minutes. Turn it once or twice with wooden spoons. Drain the spinach. Measure 1 cup and serve as is or chopped well. Serving ideas: Top with allowable portion of melted butter, lemon juice, salt, pepper, and nutmeg. Toss with allowable portion of olive oil and Parmesan cheese. Serve with hard-boiled eggs.

Ingredients

1 - 2 pounds spinach

Spinach-Artichoke Dip

Heat oven to 350°F. Spray an ovenproof pan with Pam or zero-calorie butter spray. In a food processor, process spinach, artichokes, garlic, ricotta cheese, Parmesan, and pepper until well combined, scraping down sides of processor, as needed. Spread mixture in prepared pan. Bake until warmed through, about 30 minutes. Serve hot with sliced vegetables. Makes 1 cooked vegetable and 1 protein.

Ingredients

3 ounces ricotta cheese ◆ 1/2 ounce grated Parmesan cheese ◆ 1/2 cup frozen chopped spinach, thawed ◆ 1/2 cup artichoke bottoms ◆ 2 cloves garlic ◆ 1/4 teaspoon freshly ground pepper

Squash Chips

Cut both ends off the squash with a cleaver, then use a small paring knife to remove the skin. Cut off the bottom of the squash and remove seeds. Slice squash into very thin half-circles and spread in a single layer on baking sheets. Sprinkle with salt and seasoning. Bake at 450° for about 15 minutes, taking care not to burn squash slices. It takes quite a stack to make 8 ounces.

Ingredients

1 large butternut squash ◆ seasoning mix of your choice—I like Mexican ones myself ◆ salt

Squash with Four Chiles

Bake the squash for about an hour at 400° F or microwave until tender. Slice in half and leave to cool. Soak the chipotle in boiling water for 5 minutes and drain. Pulverize the ancho in a blender or food processor. Stem and seed the habañero. Place all three chiles in a large pot with 1 cup water. Simmer 20 minutes; remove and discard chipotle and habañero. Scrape squash from rind; whirl in blender or food processor and add to pot.Simmer 10 minutes. Meanwhile, sauté the jalapeños and onions in the oil. When they are finished, add them to the squash and mix thoroughly.

Ingredients

2 large butternut squashl ◆3 lb banana squashl ◆1 dried chipotle pepperl ◆1 dried ancho chilel ◆1 fresh habañero or other hot pepperl ◆1 small red onion finely choppedl ◆2-3 jalapeño peppers roasted and choppedl ◆ 1 Tb olive oi

Squash with Herbs and Spices

Peel and cut the squash into pieces. Put in a pan with water, and simmer until just tender. Remove squash from pan. Add spices to the liquid, which remains, bring to a boil, return squash to pan, and simmer until squash is very soft.

Ingredients

1 medium-sized squash ◆ 1/2 teaspoon ground pepper ◆ 1/4 teaspoon ground cumin ◆ 1/4 teaspoon ground ginger ◆ pinch of rosemary ◆ 1 tablespoon cider vinegar

Steamed asparagus with Cheese

Wash fresh asparagus. Cut tips and main part. Discard last 2 inches of stem. Steam in large bowl for 8 minutes in microwave or on stove. Measure 2 ozs. Velveeta cheese or Cheezewiz or other hard cheese. Slice in small chunks to cover steamed asparagus. Cover. Let sit 5 to 10 minutes until cheese is melted.

Ingredients

8 to 16 oz. Fresh asparagus ◆ 2 oz. Velveeta or CheezWiz or other hard cheese

Steamed Asparagus with Texas Best BBQ Sauce (Blue Label)

I love this vegetable. Sometimes I cook 4 bundles at a time and marinate some in balsamic vinegar so it keeps a long time. The Texas Best is only abstinent in the "Original Recipe" version (blue label).

Stir Fry

Spray pan with butter spray generously. Stir fry green onions, red and yellow bell peppers and spinach at the end.

Ingredients

Green Onions ◆ Red and Yellow Bell Peppers ◆ spinach

Stir-Fried Veggies

Heat some oil and add the thinly sliced veggies one at a time. Cook until soft but still crunchy and slight seared. Season to taste. I then weigh out my portions and keep them in boxes for the next few days and I always have a vegetable side dish available when I need it.

Ingredients

Carrots ◆ Zucchini ◆ Cabbage ◆ Asparagus ◆ Mushrooms ◆ Salt ◆ Pepper ◆ Tabasco Sauce (I like spicy!!) ◆ Peanut Oil for Frying (or any other that you like and/or are allowed)

String Beans

Take about 1 pound raw of string beans. Clean them. Spray Pyrex dish with vegetable spray. Put the string beans in the dish. Add either fresh chopped garlic or dry powdered garlic to taste. Add about 3 tablespoons of soy sauce. generous sprinkle of sesame seeds. Toss together and microwave covered until cooked as tender as you like. I like mine crispy and not overcooked. I usually cook for about 5 minutes. Mix again then put back for another 3 minutes.

Ingredients

1 pound Raw String Beans ◆ Fresh or Powdered Chopped Garlic ◆ 3 tablespoons Soy Sauce ◆ Sesame Seeds

String Beans Egyptian Style

Wash green beans and slice them in half. Fry the onions in a large, thick-bottomed saucepan with a small amount of water until they turn soft. Add the beans, and fry very gently until they are slightly softened. Stir in the tomato paste, blending it well. Add enough water to barely cover the vegetables, then nutmeg, cinnamon, lemon juice, and salt and pepper. Stir thoroughly. Bring to a boil, cover, reduce heat, and simmer gently until vegetables are very tender and sauce very thick. Measure 1/2 cup and serve.

Ingredients

2 pounds string beans ◆ 2 large onions ◆ finely chopped ◆ 3 tablespoons tomato paste ◆ 1/4 teaspoon nutmeg ◆ 1/2 teaspoon cinnamon ◆ 2 tablespoons lemon juice ◆ salt and pepper

String Beans in Garlic Sauce

Trim ends off beans and cut in half. In one bowl, combine garlic and chili paste. In another bowl, mix soy sauce, vinegar, and sweetener. Heat wok sprayed heavily with zero-calorie cooking spray over medium heat. Add the green beans and stir-fry until they begin to brown. Remove to a bowl. Add scallions to wok, stir-fry quickly, and remove to same bowl. Heat wok sprayed heavily with Pam again. When it is hot, add garlic/chili paste mixture. Stir for about 12 seconds, then add beans and stir to mix well. Add soy sauce mixture, and stir for a minute. May be prepared ahead and served cold. Quite hot; cut down on the chili paste if you have a low spice tolerance.

Ingredients

1 1/2 pounds fresh string beans ◆ 6 cloves garlic, pressed ◆ 2 teaspoons chili paste w/garlic or 3 tablespoons sugar-free ketchup with chili pepper and garlic powder added ◆ 1 tablespoon soy sauce ◆ 1 tablespoon vinegar ◆ 2 teaspoons liquid sweetener ◆ 1 1/2 cups diced scallions ◆ zero-calorie cooking spray

String Beans, Cooked

Wash fresh beans. Tear off the blossom end and pull down to remove any strings. Bring a pan of salted water to a rolling boil - enough to more than cover the beans. Add prepared beans in several batches in order to keep the water boiling. Cook at a rolling boil a few minutes, then reduce the heat to medium and cook slowly 12 to 15 minutes. Drain the beans at once. To serve cold, plunge in cold water and drain again. To serve hot, dry out the pan in which they were cooked by putting over medium heat for a moment. Add beans and let them reheat briefly before adding allowable portion of butter and seasonings. Shake the pan to prevent scorching. String beans may also be steamed for 12-14 minutes. If beans are limp, freshen them in plastic bag in refrigerator drawer.

Ingredients

1 - 2 pounds string beans ◆ butter

String Beans, Roasted

Heat oven to 375° F. In a large bowl, spray zero-calorie butter spray on green beans and salt. Toss to coat. Spread out beans in a single layer on 2 pans. Roast beans 20 minutes, until lightly browned and crisp-tender. Flip beans halfway through cooking time for even browning. Measure 1 cup and serve.

Ingredients

3 pounds thin green beans
◆ zero-calorie butter spray (olive oil flavored) ◆ 3/4 teaspoon salt

Stuffing

Cook onions and celery in Pam until soft. Add mushrooms. Set aside. Add broth to water. Add to TVP. Add vegetables. Use a little stiffly beaten egg white to hold it all together.

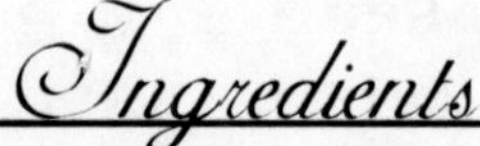

1 oz. TVP ◆ 1/4 cup chopped cooked onions, celery, & mushrooms
◆ 1 c boiled water ◆ Garlic Pam ◆ egg white
◆ powdered chicken broth or onion soup ◆ garlic
◆ seasonings you like

Summer Squash Sautee

Spray zero-calorie butter spray in large pan. Add zucchini, squash, green beans, and garlic. Cook until desired consistency. Measure 1 cup and serve. Variation: Add 1/4 cup onion, finely chopped, with other vegetables, and measure 1/2 cup serving.

Ingredients

2 medium zucchini sliced into 1/2 inch strips ◆ 2 medium yellow summer squash sliced into 1/2 inch strips ◆ fresh string beans (a few handfuls) ◆ 2 cloves garlic - finely chopped ◆ zero-calorie butter spray (olive flavor is good)

Summer Squash, Grilled with Basil

Prepare a medium grill or heat broiler. In a large bowl, combine zucchini, yellow squash, allowable portion of oil, salt and pepper. Toss to coat. Grill squash (in batches, if necessary) 2 to 3 minutes per side until lightly charred and just tender. Transfer to a large bowl and toss with basil, parsley, lemon juice, lemon rind. Measure 1 cup and serve.

Ingredients

2 medium zucchini summer squash, trimmed and cut diagonally into 1/4" slices ◆ 1 medium yellow summer squash, trimmed and cut diagonally into 1/4" slices ◆ olive oil ◆ 1/2 teaspoon salt ◆ 1/4 teaspoon pepper ◆ 3 tb thinly sliced basil leaves ◆ 1 tb chopped fresh parsley ◆ 2 teaspoons fresh lemon juice

Summer Squash, Sautéed

Cut squash in rounds or long fingers. Sauté quickly in skillet with zero-calorie butter spray. Season with finely chopped garlic clove, salt, and pepper. Squash is done when it is just tender but still firm. Do not overcook. Measure 1 cup and serve. Serving ideas: Top with allowable portion of butter, olive oil, and/or lemon juice.

Ingredients

1 pound summer squash, or zucchini ◆ zero-calorie butter spray

Summer Squash, Steamed

Slice squash in rounds, strips, quarters, or lengthwise. Drop into boiling, salted water in heavy saucepan. Steam covered until just crisply tender. Drain. Measure 1 cup and serve with allowable portion of butter and/or lemon juice.

Ingredients

1 - 2 pounds summer squash, or zucchini ◆ salt ◆ butter ◆ lemon juice

Sun-Dried Tomatoes

Slice the tomatoes in half vertically, remove seeds, and place face-up on baking sheets. Sprinkle with salt and bake at 400° for 15 minutes. Lower heat to 225° and bake for another 2 1/2 hours; check them after about 2 hours to make sure the bottoms have not burned. When tomatoes are small, shriveled things, put them in plastic containers and add garlic and basil. Cover with olive oil. Seal the containers and freeze until ready to use. May be refrozen; they'll keep all winter.

Ingredients

Buckets of fresh flavorful Roma tomatoes ◆ salt ◆ fresh basil ◆ fresh garlic ◆ olive oil

Sweet and Sour Onions

Bring 3 quarts of water to a boil; drop in the onions, count to 15, and drain. As soon as they are cool enough to handle, pull off the outside skin, detach any roots, and cut a cross into the butt end. Place onions in a sauté pan which will hold them without overlapping. Add butter and enough water to come no more than 1 inch up the sides of the pan. Turn the heat on to medium and cook, adding water whenever the liquid in the pan becomes insufficient. In 20 minutes or so, when the onions begin to soften, add the vinegar, sweetener, salt, and pepper, and turn the heat down to low. Continue to cook for 1 hour or more, adding water whenever it becomes necessary. Onions are done when they become colored a rich, dark golden brown all over, and are easily pierced with a fork.

Ingredients

3 lbs small white boiling Onions ◆ 1 tablespoons Butter ◆ 3 tablespoons Cider Cinegar ◆ 2 teaspoons liquid Sweetener ◆ Salt and Black Pepper

Sweet and Sour Squash

Soften squash in microwave; peel and cut into cubes, discarding seeds. Heat the oil in a shallow pan. Add fenugreek, cumin, fennel, and mustard seeds and cook until browned. Add curry leaves, green chilis, red pepper, and asafetida; stir. Add squash, ginger, turmeric, and salt; mix well and cook covered until squash softens (you may need to add a little water). Remove cover; add coriander, chili powder, and amchoor. Mix and add sweetener. Cook on medium heat about 15 minutes. Add tamarind, stir well, and serve hot.

Ingredients

2 acorn squash ◆ 1 teaspoon tamarind paste ◆ 2 whole green chilis, chopped ◆ 2 inch piece of ginger peeled and chopped ◆ 1 whole dried red pepper ◆ 5-10 curry leaves (optional) ◆ 1/2 teaspoon fenugreek seeds ◆ 1/2 teaspoon cumin seeds ◆ 1/2 teaspoon mustard seeds ◆ 1 teaspoon fennel seeds ◆ 2 pinches asafetida ◆ 1/2 teaspoon turmeric ◆ 1 teaspoon salt ◆ 2 teaspoon ground coriander ◆ 1 teaspoon red chili powder ◆ 1 teaspoon liquid sweetener ◆ 1 tablespoon vegetable oil

Tofu Cacciatore

To squeeze excess moisture from tofu, place tofu slices on a baking sheet. Cover with parchment paper or plastic wrap and set a second baking sheet on top. Place weights (heavy cans or pans) on top of the baking sheet. Set aside for 15 minutes. (Or, if you want a meatier texture, spread tofu slices on a baking sheet, cover with plastic wrap and freeze until ready to use.) Preheat oven to 350 degrees F (175 degrees C). Spray a saute pan once with cooking spray and place pan over low heat. Add peppers and cook, stirring frequently, for 5 minutes. Add garlic, basil, and oregano and cook, stirring, for 15 seconds. Stir in tomatoes and tomato paste. Cover and simmer for 15 minutes. While sauce is simmering, spray a large sauté pan or griddle once with cooking spray and place pan over low heat. Brown the tofu in the pan lightly on both sides. Measure 4 ounces tofu and 8 ounces cooked vegetables. Individual servings can be placed in Pyrex baking cups. Cover tofu with tomato-pepper sauce. Cover baking cups with parchment paper and aluminum foil. Bake for 30 - 45 minutes -- the longer they bake, the more flavor the tofu will absorb. Variations: 1 medium onion may be added with peppers on maintenance. If allowed, use 1/2 portion of cooked vegetable to stir-fry tofu in wheat germ, and use other 1/2 portion cooked vegetable to cover tofu with tomato-pepper sauce.

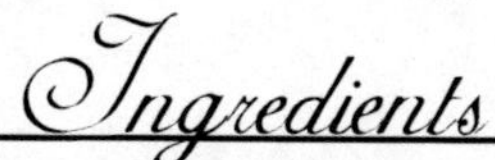

2 pounds firm tofu, cut into 1/2 inch thick slices ◆ 2 bell peppers, cored and sliced ◆ 3 5-ounce cans chopped tomatoes, drained ◆ 2 tablespoons tomato paste ◆ 1 tablespoon finely chopped fresh garlic ◆ 2 teaspoons dried basil ◆ 2 teaspoons dried oregano ◆ zero-calorie butter spray ◆ salt ◆ pepper

Tomato Puree

Mix ingredients together well. Heat in Micro wave. Can add mbt or bouillon if you use it.

Ingredients

2 oz tomato paste ◆ salt ◆ dash of sweet low ◆ pepper ◆ water

Tomato Sauce

Combine ingredients and add water to desired consistency.

Ingredients

2 oz tomato paste ◆ salt ◆ (oil measured per meal plan optional and not necessary) ◆ Pepper ◆ drops of Louisiana (or any) hot sauce ◆ Dash of oregano(dry)

Tomato Sauce "Honeymoon"

Turn down to medium low and simmer for 5 minutes.

Ingredients

1 28 oz can Pastene ground tomatoes ◆ 3-4 stalks fresh basil ◆ whole leaves ◆ 1/4 c extra virgin olive oil ◆ 3-4 cloves garlic chopped ◆ 1 tsp salt ◆ 1 tsp peppe ◆ 1/4 - 1/2 tsp red pepper flakes

Tomato, Baked

Preheat oven to 350F and spray a baking pan with cooking spray. Place the tomatoes cut side up on the pan and sprinkle evenly with the black pepper, garlic powder, parmesan and then the oregano. Preheat oven to 350F and spray a baking pan with cooking spray. Place the tomatoes cut side up on the pan and sprinkle evenly with the black pepper, garlic powder, parmesan and then the oregano.

Ingredients

1/2 ounce parmesan cheese ◆ 2 large ripe but firm tomatoes, cut in half ◆ 1 teaspoon oregano ◆ 1/4 teaspoon fresh ground black pepper ◆ 1/2 teaspoon garlic powder ◆ zero-calorie cooking spray

Tomatoes with Onion and Basil

Heat oil in a heavy-bottomed pan and add onions, garlic, and red pepper flakes. Sauté until onions are soft and golden. Add tomatoes and stir frequently to help them break down. Add salt and basil leaves when tomatoes start to look done. Continue to cook over high heat until you have a thick sauce like mixture

Ingredients

1 Tb extra-virgin olive oil ◆ 3 cloves garlic peeled and diced ◆ 2 medium onions diced ◆ pinch of red pepper flakes ◆ 2 cans chopped tomatoes or 1 lb good fresh ripe Roma tomatoes quartered ◆ 6 large fresh basil leaves ◆ salt to taste

Tomatoes with Onion and Basil

Heat oil in a heavy-bottomed pan and add onions, garlic, and red pepper flakes. Sauté until onions are soft and golden. Add tomatoes and stir frequently to help them break down. Add salt and basil leaves when tomatoes start to look done. Continue to cook over high heat until you have a thick sauce like mixture

Ingredients

1 Tb extra-virgin olive oil ◆ 3 cloves garlic peeled and diced ◆ 2 medium onions diced ◆ pinch of red pepper flakes ◆ 2 cans chopped tomatoes or 1 lb good fresh ripe Roma tomatoes quartered ◆ 6 large fresh basil leaves ◆ salt to taste

Tomatoes, Broiled Sicilian Style

Remove tops of tomatoes and rub tomatoes with salt. Squeeze lightly to loosen the pulp, and turn onto absorbent paper. Combine seasonings and whirl in a grinder or pound in a mortar. Spray heavy skillet with zero-calorie butter spray. Add seasonings to skillet. Place tomatoes cut side down in mixture. Simmer over medium-low heat about 30 minutes, till tomatoes are cooked through. Stop before mushy or overdone. Turn tomatoes back upright and spoon pan juices over them. Measure 1 cup and serve. These can be found on menus in New York and California. They are unusually good.

Ingredients

6 quite firm ripe tomatoes ◆ zero-calorie butter spray ◆ 1/2 teaspoon allspice ◆ 1 teaspoon cinnamon ◆ 3 garlic cloves, finely chopped ◆ 1/4 cup chopped parsley ◆ 1 teaspoon dry basil or 1 tablespoon chopped fresh basil ◆ 1 teaspoon salt ◆ 1/2 teaspoon freshly ground pepper

Tomatoes, Peeled

Drop tomatoes in boiling water for a moment, and remove them at once, or hold tomatoes over gas flame for moment or two, turning them until the skin pops. If the skin appears to be coarse, a tomato is better peeled.

Ingredients

Tomatoes

Tomatoes, Stewed

Peel tomatoes by scalding for a moment in water or roasting over flame until skin pops. Spray heavy skillet with zero-calorie butter spray. Add tomatoes. Cook slowly, covered, until they break down. Add salt and sweetener and continue cooking about 10 minutes. Measure 1 cup and serve. Variations: Add 2 tablespoons chopped basil. Add 1/2 cup finely chopped onion (reducing a serving to 1/2 cup). Add 1 finely chopped garlic clove. Add 1 tablespoon lemon juice. Add 3 canned, peeled green chilies, finely chopped.

Ingredients

4 pounds tomatoes ◆ zero-calorie butter spray ◆ salt ◆ pepper ◆ 1 teaspoon sweetener

Tuna Melt

Put 1/8 cup wheat germ at bottom of plastic container. Mix with 1/4 cup water, and microwave for 4-6 minutes, until it looks like a crust. Mix allowable portion of mayonnaise with tuna. Top the wheat germ with tuna mixture, sliced tomato, and sliced cheese. Broil or microwave until the cheese melts.

Ingredients

2 ounces tuna ◆ 1 ounce sliced, or shredded cheese ◆ 1/8 cup wheat germ ◆ 1 sliced tomato (from Finger Salad at Lunch or from Salad at Dinner) ◆ mayonnaise

Turnip Fries

Heat oven to 425° F. Cut turnips into 2" x 1/2" sticks. Place on a foil-lined pan. Spray with zero-calorie butter spray. Sprinkle with salt and chili powder. Turn with spatula to coat. Spread out in a single layer. Roast fries 30 minutes, turning halfway through cooking time for even browning. Measure 1 cup and serve.

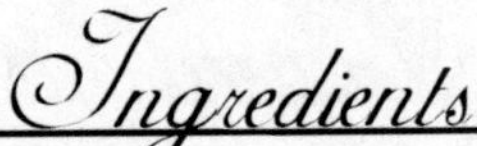

4 turnips, trimmed and peeled (about 1 1/4 pounds) ◆ zero-calorie butter spray (olive oil flavored) ◆ 1 teaspoon salt ◆ 1/2 teaspoon chili powder

Turnip Recipe

Spray pan with non stick spray and mix all vegetables. Bake uncovered for 35 minutes (or until all veggies are tender) at 350-375 Measure and add your fat (olive oil is the best, but butter is tasty too)

Ingredients

Turnip (or rutabaga) cut up ◆ 3-4 whole carrots in 3" slices ◆ 2 big (Spanish or Vidalia) onions in quarters ◆ 4 sprigs of fresh rosemary ◆ salt and pepper to taste

Turnip Vegetable Casserole

Cut all vegetables into 1/2 inch slices and place in a baking dish that is sprayed with non stick spray. Sprinkle with fresh rosemary, sage, salt and pepper. Roast uncovered at 350 degrees for 25 minutes. Turn slightly to make sure the vegetables brown evenly. Bake for another 15 to 20 minutes or until all vegetables are thoroughly cooked.

Ingredients

1 turnip ◆ 2 carrots ◆ 2 onions ◆ 10 brussel sprouts ◆ fresh rosemary ◆ sage ◆ salt and pepper

Turnips "Dry" with Onions

Boil the turnips ahead of time; when they are cool enough to handle, peel and mash coarsely or dice. Heat the oil in wok or heavy skillet over medium heat. Add asafetida and let it sizzle for a few seconds. Add cumin and mustard seeds, then, after about 10 seconds, the red pepper(s). When pepper(s) darken(s), add chopped onions and turmeric. After the onions begin to brown at the edges, add turnips, salt, garam masala, and lemon juice. Fry, stirring, for 5-7 minutes. Measure and serve.

Ingredients

2 lbs turnips ◆ 1 Tb vegetable oil ◆ 1/8 tsp asafetida ◆ 1/2 tsp whole cumin seeds ◆ 2 1/2 tsp whole black mustard seeds ◆ 1-3 whole dried red peppers ◆ 1 medium onion peeled and coarsely chopped, ◆ 1/2 tsp ground turmeric ◆ 1 1/4 tsp salt ◆ 1 tsp garam masala ◆ 2 Tb lemon juice

Turnips and Carrots, Mashed

Peel skin off of the turnip then cut turnip into pieces. Size doesn't matter, but the smaller you cut them the faster they will boil. Place turnip pieces in a saucepan with water and a touch of salt and boil till done. When you can stick a fork through piece, it's done! Cut up carrots as well and boil until done. When turnip and carrot are ready, put both in one bowl or saucepan and mash them together. Or you can mash them separately and then mix them together. (A food processor can also be used.) Measure 1/2 cup and serve hot. Add salt and pepper to taste. Measure.

Ingredients

1 turnip ◆ 6 carrots ◆ salt ◆ pepper

Turnips, Boiled

Peel turnips, and cut them in even dice, rounds, or slices. Cook them in boiling, salted water for about 15 to 20 minutes, or just until tender. Drain. Measure 1 cup and serve with allowable portion of butter, salt, and pepper. Smaller turnips are more delicate in texture and flavor. Serving ideas: Add equal amount of sliced, sautéed mushrooms and 1 tablespoon finely chopped parsley. Measure 1/2 cup and serve.

Ingredients

6 to 8 small turnips ◆ salt ◆ pepper ◆ allowable portion of butter

Turnips, Stir-Fried

Mix soy sauce, sweetener, and vinegar in small bowl; set aside. Heat a wok or heavy skillet, sprayed heavily with zero-calorie cooking spray, over medium-high heat. Stir-fry the ginger, garlic, scallions, salt, and pepper about 30 seconds. Add turnips and stir-fry for 2 minutes. Stir in soy sauce mixture. Cook, stirring constantly, until sauce thickens slightly (about 2 minutes). Measure and serve.

Ingredients

3/4 pound turnips, peeled, thinly sliced, parboiled 4 minutes, and drained ◆ 2 tablespoons light soy sauce ◆ 1 teaspoon sweetener ◆ 1 tablespoon white vinegar ◆ zero-calorie cooking spray ◆ 1 teaspoon grated fresh ginger root ◆ 2 cloves garlic, minced ◆ 4 scallions, including tender green tops, minced ◆ 1/2 teaspoon salt ◆ 1 teaspoon freshly ground pepper

Vegetable Stew

Put vegetables, garlic and brown sugar in a small pot. Add 2 cups of water. Boil until tender.

Ingredients

1 cup of vegetables cut up in small pieces ◆ garlic ◆ Sweet N Low brown sugar

Vegetarian Spaghetti

Cook in microwave until warm & steamy and the flavors have had a chance to "acquaint" themselves.

Ingredients

4 oz spaghetti squash, cooked any way you choose ◆ 1 T butter or olive oil ◆ 2 oz pasta sauce ◆ 1/2 oz parmesan cheese

VOILA.... RATATOUILLE

Cover and cook for about 1 hour on very low flame (make sure to add plenty of salt and pepper). I serve it over salad or rice!

Ingredients

3 or 4 zucchini in 1 inch chunks ◆ 1 large purple onion (purple only for vitamins, any color is ok) ◆ 2 very large tomatoes or about 4 plum tomatoes ◆ 1 whole box, or about 10 mushrooms ◆ 1 green pepper

West Indian Squash

Heat oil in a Dutch oven or soup pot over medium heat. Add onions, celery, and carrots; cook until soft but not brown, 3-4 minutes. Add garlic and chiles and cook for 1 minute more. Add the squash cubes, parsley, bay leaves, thyme, and sweetener and enough water to half-cover the vegetables. Bring to a boil, then reduce heat to medium-low and simmer until the vegetables are very soft, 25-30 minutes. If there is too much liquid remaining in the pan, raise heat and boil off the excess. Discard the bay leaves and thyme sprigs before serving.

Ingredients

1 Tb olive oil ◆ 1 onion, chopped ◆ 2 stalks celery chopped ◆ 1 carrot chopped ◆ 3 cloves garlic minced ◆ 1/2 habañero seeded and finely chopped ◆ 5 cups water ◆ 1 large calabaza or butternut squash peeled seeded and cubed ◆ 1/4 cup finely chopped fresh parsley ◆ 2 bay leaves ◆ 2 sprigs fresh thyme or 1 tsp. dried thyme leaves ◆ 1 Tb liquid sweetener ◆ salt and freshly ground black pepper ◆ chopped chives for garnish ◆ 1/4 tsp. ground red pepper (cayenne) for garnish

Wheat Germ Squash Cookies

Mix ingredients together and spoon into muffin tin sprayed with abstinent cooking spray. Bake at 325 for 1/2 hour.

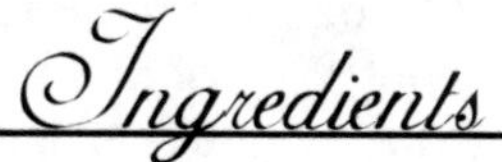

2 oz of pumpkin or Cooked acorn squash ◆ 1/4 oz wheat germ ◆ 1 Tbs. Butter ◆ 1 packet equal ◆ ginger ◆ nutmeg cinnamon to taste

Wheat Germ Coffee Cookie

Put wheat germ in small, shallow dish. Pour in your favorite flavor of coffee syrup, just enough to make moist mixture. Microwave for 1 minute, or just enough to cook without burning. These are fantastic for traveling!

Ingredients

1/8 cup wheat germ ◆ 1/8 cup alcohol-free ◆ sugar-free coffee syrup

Wheat Germ Cookie, Maintenance

Spray pan with zero-calorie butter spray. Heat stove to medium or med/low until hot. In a small bowl, or container, mix wheat germ, egg, oil, flavoring, and sweetener. Add very little water or diet cream soda, and stir. Cook on preheated pan. Turn once and enjoy. For different tastes, add almond flavor to almond oil, or vanilla and cinnamon to peanut oil or hazelnut oil. For other flavors, use vanilla and almond oil, and add a very small amount of coconut, orange. Travels great and can be frozen for future use. Takes a little time, but it's worth it. Makes 1 Cooked Vegetable, on some Maintenance plans, and 1 oz. Protein. Check with your sponsor.

Ingredients

1/4 cup wheat germ (or 1 oz.) ◆ 1 oz. Egg ◆ 1 tablespoon oil - peanut, almond, or hazelnut ◆ water or diet cream soda, ◆ 1/4 oz. extract - vanilla, almond, coconut, or cinnamon ◆ sweetener ◆ zero-calorie butter spray

White Turnip

Cut into small cubes. Boil or steam or steam or cook in microwave (at level 8 for 8 minutes)

Ingredients

White Turnip

Winter Squash Souffle

Puree cooked squash, and season as usual with salt and pepper, adding a pinch of nutmeg and cinnamon. Beat eggs in a bowl until thoroughly mixed. Spray shallow glass or foil casserole dish with zero-calorie butter spray. Pour beaten eggs into baking dish. Fold in squash until mixed with eggs. Bake at 350 degrees for 25 minutes, or until nicely puffed and browned.

Ingredients

2 eggs ◆ 1/2 cup winter squash ◆ zero-calorie butter spray ◆ salt ◆ pepper ◆ cinnamon ◆ nutmeg

Winter Squash, Baked

Cut winter squash in half lengthwise. Remove seeds and clean thoroughly. Spray halves liberally with zero-calorie butter spray. Top with seasonings. Bake in oven at 375 F, either in a pan of water or on the rack. Cook 30 - 45 minutes. (Hubbard squash may take 1 hour.) When tender, scoop meat out from shells. Surprisingly, winter squash is also good chilled, after cooking, served with yogurt!

Ingredients

1 winter squash (Acorn, Butternut, Danish, Hubbard, Nutmeg, Turban) ◆ zero-calorie butter spray, abstinent seasonings

Winter Squash, Butternut

Cut in half lengthwise. Remove seeds. Place on shallow, microwave-safe dish, skin side up. Add small amount of water to bottom of dish. Cover with lid. Microwave for 15-20 minutes, depending on size of squash. Cool for 10 minutes. Scoop out meat. Measure 1/2 cup and serve hot or chilled. Serving ideas: Serve hot, topped with measured cheese. Serve cold, mixed with yogurt, sweetener, and abstinent flavorings.

Ingredients

1 butternut winter squash

Winter Squash, Butternut Chips

Cut both ends off the squash with a cleaver; then use a small paring knife to remove the skin. Cut off the bottom of the squash and remove seeds. Slice squash into very thin half-circles and spread in a single layer on baking sheets. Sprinkle with fajita seasoning (or salt, pepper, other spices of your choice). Bake at 450°F for about 15 minutes, taking care not to burn squash slices. Measure 1/2 cup portion and serve. This works with other kinds of squash, though not as well, and with rutabagas and turnips. May also be cooked in the oven broiler.

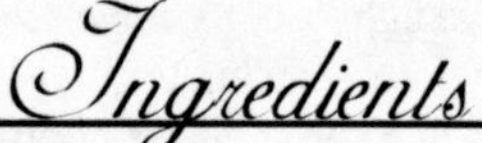

1 large butternut winter squash ◆ fajita seasoning or chili powder and onion salt

Winter Squash, Spaghetti

Heat oven to 400 F. Prick squash in several places and bake 45 minutes until tender. Allow to cool slightly. Cut in half, lengthwise, and scoop out seeds. Pull out squash strands from each side with a fork. Transfer to a container for storage. Measure 1/2 cup and serve hot or cold.

Ingredients

1 whole spaghetti winter squash

Winter Squash, Spaghetti a la Gorgonzola

Split spaghetti squash lengthwise and remove seeds. Place flat side of squash down in a microwave dish with about ½ inch water and cover. Cook on high for approximately 15-30 minutes. (Squash is done when tender but not mushy to the touch.) Loosen strands with a fork. Measure out 1/2 cup of the cooked squash. Add remaining ingredients, and microwave until cheese and butter are melted (about 2 minutes). Top with additional zero calorie butter spray, if desired.

Ingredients

1 whole spaghetti winter squash ◆ 1 1/2 ounces gorgonzola or bleu cheese ◆ 1/2 ounce Parmesan or Romano cheese ◆ butter ◆ salt and pepper

Winter Squash, Spaghetti Hawaiian Style

Toss squash with butter, cinnamon, and sweetener. Top with ham and soy nuts. Add additional zero calorie butter spray, if desired.

Ingredients

3 ounces cooked diced ham ◆ 1 ounce soy nuts ◆ 1/2 cup spaghetti winter squash, butter or margarine ◆ 1/2 teaspoon cinnamon (more or less, to taste) ◆ sweetener

Yellow Squash Frittata

Toss squash with butter, cinnamon, and sweetener. Top with ham and soy nuts. Add additional zero calorie butter spray, if desired.

Ingredients

2 - 3 yellow summer squash ◆ 1 egg ◆ 1 ounce cheese, grated ◆ Italian seasoning ◆ zero-calorie butter spray ◆ salt and pepper

Zesty Zucchini Italian Meal

Measure out 1 cup of cooked zucchini mix. Add the browned tofu to the zucchini mix and mix in ½ cup of tomato sauce. Adjust seasonings. Top with mozzarella.

Ingredients

mozzarella ◆ zucchini

Zucchini

I put a tablespoon of lemon juice in skillet on medium to med high heat, and put zucchini cut in thin long julienne strips in skillet and stir fry crisp, adding lemon pepper, and onion salt, then when just about done, I added tomato's cut in bite size pieces, for just a few minutes. (May have to add a bit of water as it cooks). Then remove, and weigh out 8 ounces of vegetables (could add onion or any other fresh vegetables to stir fry). Then I added my 1 teaspoon butter, and 1/4 ounce of grated parmesan cheese (I could still have 3 1/2 ounces of protein).

Ingredients

Zucchini ◆ 1 tablespoon Lemon Juice ◆ Lemon Pepper ◆ Onion ◆ Salt ◆ Tomato ◆ 1 teasponn Butter ◆ 1/4 oz. grated Parmesan Cheese

Zucchini Broiled with Parmesan Cheese

2 ounces grated Parmesan cheese, 1 cup zucchini summer squash, thinly sliced longways, in fan shapes, zero-calorie butter spray (olive oil flavored), 1/2 teaspoon salt, 1/4 teaspoon pepper Broil about 6 minutes or until zucchini is softened. Carefully spread fans out more. Sprinkle with cheese. Broil 5 to 6 minutes more, until cheese is lightly browned.

Ingredients

2 ounces grated Parmesan cheese ◆ 1 cup zucchini summer squash, thinly sliced longways, in fan shapes ◆ zero-calorie butter spray (olive oil flavored) ◆ 1/2 teaspoon salt ◆ 1/4 teaspoon pepper

Zucchini, Sauteed

Cut zucchini into thin strips. Spray heavy skillet with zero-calorie butter spray. Add zucchini strips. Saute lightly, turning them once or twice, for 5 minutes. Add garlic, salt, and basil. Cover the pan, and simmer for about 10 minutes, until just tender. Add the pepper. Measure 1 cup and serve. Serving ideas: After adding garlic and basil, add 1/2 cup tomato sauce, cover and simmer 10 minutes. Use part of measured protein to sprinkle zucchini with grated Parmesan cheese.

Ingredients

3 or 4 small zucchini cut in quarters lengthwise ◆ zero-calorie butter spray ◆ 1 clove finely chopped garlic ◆ 1/2 teaspoon salt ◆ 1 teaspoon chopped fresh basil ◆ 1/4 teaspoon freshly ground pepper ◆ 1 tablespoon chopped parsley

Broccoli Souffle

Puree, or finely chop, cooked broccoli. Beat eggs in a bowl until thoroughly mixed. Spray shallow glass or foil casserole dish with zero-calorie butter spray Pour beaten eggs into baking dish. Fold in broccoli until mixed with eggs. Puree, or finely chop, cooked broccoli. Beat eggs in a bowl until thoroughly mixed. Spray shallow glass or foil casserole dish with zero-calorie butter spray Pour beaten eggs into baking dish. Fold in broccoli until mixed with eggs.

Ingredients

2 eggs ◆ 1 cup broccoli ◆ zero-calorie butter spray ◆ salt, pepper

Anchovy-beet-spaghetti squash

Cook spaghetti squash. Boil beets and grate them. Sautee shallots or garlic in olive oil. Throw in the spaghetti squash w/olive oil and then mix with the grated beets. Top w/ parmesan cheese and 1/2- 1 oz anchovy.

Ingredients

3/4 cup spaghetti squash ◆ 1/4 cup cooked and grated beets, shallots or garlic ◆ olive oil ◆ parmesan cheese ◆ 1/2 to 1 oz. anchovy

Barbara's Antipasto Salad

Bake pepperoni in microwave for 2-3 minutes until light and crispy. Mix vegetables, soynuts, pepperoni, and wheat germ together. Sprinkle with onion or garlic powder. Mix dressing ingredients up right on the salad.

Ingredients

pepperoni ◆ Mix vegetables ◆ soynuts ◆ pepperon ◆ wheat germ

Abstinent Pizza

Put the dough on the pan and put in the oven on the center rack. After 10 minutes remove from the oven, turn, and apply the tomatoe sauce and the cheese. Cook for 10 more minutes and

Ingredients

3 oz soy flour ◆ 1 tsp garlic powder ◆ 1/2 tsp salt ◆ 2 oz tomato sauce ◆ 1/2 oz grated cheese ◆ 1/4 c warm water ◆ Non stick cooking spray ◆ 1 tsp onion powder ◆ 1 tsp Italian seasonings. Variation ◆ 1 oz tofu cheese

Cooked Vegetable with Protein

Cauliflower AuGratin

Mash up cooked vegetables and add remaining ingredients.

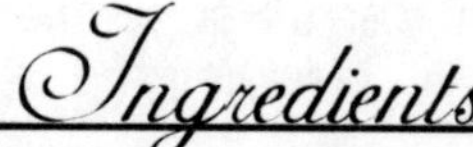

1 head fresh cauliflower ◆ Olive Oil ◆ Grated Parmesan Cheese

Butternut Squash Latkes

Mix together the first 8 ingredients Heat up frying pan till just hot. Spray pan with cooking spray (if using oil, add oil). Drop by tablespoon into pan.

Ingredients

2 eggs ◆ 1 cup broccoli ◆ zero-calorie butter spray ◆ salt ◆ pepper

CARROT LOAF/PUMPKIN/ZUCCHINI

Mash up cooked vegetables and add remaining ingredients.

Ingredients

1 Egg ◆ 2 oz soya powder ◆ 1 tsp. Cinnamon ◆ 1/4 – 1/2 tsp nutmeg ◆ 1/2 tsp. Fresh ginger ◆ 1 tsp. cinnamon ◆ 1/4 - 1/2 tsp. nutmeg ◆ 1/2 tsp. fresh ginger,little salt ◆ sweetener ◆ vanilla (or walnut or blackberry)

Cauliflower or Broccoli Kugel

Cook cauliflower and/or broccoli in microwave or steam. (Either buy it cut and chopped already, or cut it up and partially mash with a masher after it is cooked.) Drain well. Add onion soup mix and mix well. Add slightly beaten eggs and allowable portion of mayonnaise and mix. Pour into a plate or pan, sprayed with zero-calorie butter spray. Sprinkle with paprika. Bake at 350 F for 45 minutes.

Ingredients

2 eggs ◆ 1 cup cauliflower and/or broccoli ◆ 1/2 - 1 tablespoon onion soup mix ◆ mayonnaise ◆ zero-calorie butter spray ◆ paprika

Cheryl and Karen's Spinach Pie

Frozen spinach is the easiest: nuke it 'til it's done and then weigh out four ounces. Beat egg in a straight-sided plastic container; add wheat germ, salt, pepper, and the spices of your choice. Add spinach and cheese. (Karen likes to use feta cheese for this.) Top with butter. Microwave for about 4 minutes.

Ingredients

1 Egg ◆ 1 oz. Cheese ◆ 2 tablespoons Wheat Germ ◆ 4 oz. Spinach ◆ Salt ◆ Pepper ◆ 1 teaspoon Butter

Cheryl's Pumpkin Soufflé

Melt 1 tablespoon butter in a deep, straight-sided bowl (you know, a soufflé pan), or a good-sized Rubbermaid™ container. Beat in the eggs. Beat in pumpkin, wheat germ, and spices. Microwave 5-6 minutes on high and watch it rise. Melt remaining tablespoon of butter on top.

Ingredients

2 eggs ◆ 4 oz canned pumpkin ◆ 2 tablespoon wheat germ ◆ 2 tablespoon butter, ◆ cinnamon ◆ allspice ◆ ginger ◆ sweetener

Cheryl's Pumpkin Waffles

Preheat waffle iron. Combine ingredients thoroughly in a large bowl. Pour into waffle iron and heat 'til done.

Ingredients

1 Egg ◆ 2 oz Soy Flour ◆ 4 oz Canned Pumpkin ◆ 2 tablespoon Wheat Germ ◆ 1 teaspoon Butter melted ◆ 1/2 teaspoon Cinnamon ◆ 1/4 teaspoon Salt ◆ 1/4 teaspoon Ground Ginger ◆ 1/4 teaspoon Nutmeg ◆ 1/8 teaspoon Ground Cloves

Chicken with Spinach, Garlic, and Tomato Sauce

Grill chicken breasts for 5 minutes on each side, until cooked through but not dry. Meanwhile, lightly brown the garlic in a nonstick skillet, sprayed with zero-calorie butter spray, over medium-high heat. Add the spinach and cook, tossing gently, just until leaves are wilted. Add the tomatoes, soy sauce, and vinegar. Toss well until coated and thoroughly heated. Weigh 4 ounces of chicken. Measure 1 cup of spinach and tomatoes. Place spinach and tomatoes on top of cooked chicken, and serve.

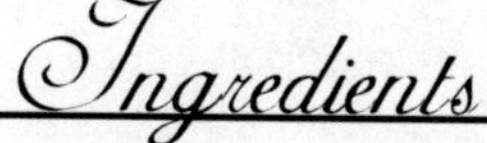

4 boneless skinless chicken breast halves (about 2 pounds total) ◆ 6 cups washed loosely packed spinach (about 1 1/2 pounds) ◆ 1 cup plum tomatoes ◆ 8-12 cloves garlic, minced ◆ 2 teaspoons soy sauce ◆ 1/4 cup vinegar ◆ zero-calorie butter spray

Eggplant & Pepperoni Parmesan

Take eggplant and slice longwise to make thin strips. Measure out 1 1/2 c eggplant and cook for a few minutes in microwave until soft. Pour off liquid. Re-measure eggplant to make 1 c or 8 ozs. and cover with pepperoni, tomato sauce and mozzarella. Bake at 350 for 10-15-20 minutes. This may also be made substituting chicken, or substituting 1/2 oz parmesan and 1/2 mozzarella for the 1 oz cheese.

Ingredients

Eggplant ◆ 1 oz mozzarella cheese ◆ 2 ozs pepperoni (it should be a brand that has dextrose listed 5th or higher as an ingredient) ◆ tomato sauce allotment

Eggplant Bake

Peel eggplant, cut through in large flat slices (do not quarter or halve); salt thoroughly and let sit overnight with a weight on top to remove thebitterness and all the liquid that comes out. Lay out on baking sheet and roast in oven until nice and dark, and pretty dry.Weigh eight ounces, serve with measured ricotta cheese (or you can serve with thick yogurt), and 2 oz tomato sauce.

Ingredients

Eggplant ◆ 8 ounces ricotta cheese or thick yogurt ◆ 2 ounces tomato sauce

Eggplant Parmesan

Slice eggplant as thin as you can. Lay slices on baking sheets (1 layer only) and sprinkle with ample amounts of paprika, curry, and salt. Drizzle oil over slices, making sure every slice has enough oil.

Ingredients

Eggplant ◆ paprika ◆ curry ◆ salt ◆ oil pasta sauce ◆ basil ◆ hard cheese

Eggplant Pizza

Slice a raw eggplant length wise in to 3/8 inch thick slices. Fry in fry pan with pan spray until tender crisp, about 3 minutes on each side. Weigh out 8 oz, place on baking sheet, close together to form the base of your pizza. Spread\ on the tomato sauce. (Hint: you can simmer a can or two of tomato sauce before hand for an hour or two with spices of your choice. I use parsley, rosemary, lots of garlic, salt and pepper. I freeze the extra sauce in 2 tablespoon batches for future use in ice trays to freeze. When frozen, pop out each 'tomato cube' into individual plastic bags and keep in freezer- so easy to grab one when you need one.) Sprinkle on the 1 oz of mozzarella and cover with 2 oz pepperoni. Bake at 375 for about 10 minutes.

Ingredients

8 oz cooked eggplant ◆ 2 oz pepperoni ◆ 1 oz mozzarella ◆ 2 tablespoons Tomato sauce

Eggplant with Ricotta and Tomato sauce

Slice eggplant thinly. Spray with Pam, sprinkle with garlic powder, oregano, basil the works. Lay on a cookie sheet or foil. Turn on the broiler of your oven, place in the oven or better yet the broiler at the very bottom of the stove. Check to make sure it not burning.Remove it, place in a bowl. Measure the ricotta and tomato sauce. Mix together...eat.

Ingredients

Eggplant ◆ Pam ◆ Garlic Powder ◆ Oregano ◆ Basil ◆ Tomato ◆ Sauce ◆ Ricotta Cheese

Faux Vegetarian Lasagna

Saute then measure the zucchini and onion in the olive oil. In a microwave safe dish, make one layer of zucchini, then add the onion, the pasta sauce, then the feta cheese, & the remainder of the zucchini. Microwave for 90 seconds, or until the cheese starts to melt and you can see steam rising.

Ingredients

6 oz zucchini, sliced ◆ 1 oz onion, chopped ◆ 1 T olive oil, seasoned with S&P and oregano ◆ 2 oz spaghetti sauce ◆ 2 oz feta cheese, cut in cubes, or crumbled.

Ham Salad

Combine ham, celery, green onions, and chopped pickles. Bind with allowable portion of mayonnaise and mustard. Arrange on greens and top with tomatoes.

Ingredients

4 ounces diced cold ham ◆ 1/2 cup lettuce greens ◆ 1/2 cup finely chopped celery ◆ 1/2 cup finely cut green onions ◆ 1/4 cup chopped tomatoes ◆ 1/4 cup finely chopped pickles ◆ mayonnaise ◆ mustard

Homemade Beef-Vegetable Soup-Stew

Place 5 cups water in a large pot of 3 qt. saucepan. Boil the beef piece slowly in the water for 15 to 20 minutes. When beef is almost cooked, add 1/4 cup quality tomato sauce to the beef broth cooking. Continue to simmer. Meanwhile, wash, clean, pare, cut and weigh vegetables to equal 16 ozs. (2 cups vegetable.). Remove beef from beef-tomato stock. Set aside to cool a bit. Place prepared vegetables in beef-tomato stock to cook for 15 to 20 minutes. Meanwhile, cut beef into small pieces. Weigh beef to measure 4 ozs. Put beef pieces back in with the vegetable-tomato-beef stock. Add 1 cup extra water if stock has boiled down. Cook an additional 5 minutes.

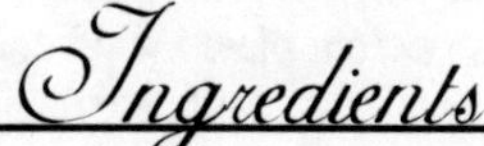

4 oz. beef (no bone) ◆ 5 cups water ◆ 1/4 cup quality tomato sauce ◆ 8 ozs. fresh green beans ◆ 6 ozs. fresh green pepper ◆ 2 ozs. red Spanish onion

Individual Pan Pizza

Cook down veggies to make 8 oz drained. Drizzle small amount of your desired/legal tom sauce over veggies with spice to taste. I dot with sweetener as well. Shred or slice thinly and dot with cheese. Cook in microwave at least 3 minutes until cheese is well melted.

Ingredients

Black pepper ◆ hot sauce ◆ oregano ◆ Diced Tomato, red (or green) pepper sliced ◆ mushrooms ◆ 2 ozs any legal firm cheese

Italian Casserole

Wash squash and put in a cellophane bag (like you get your veggies in at the grocer's). Prick the squash with a fork several times through the plastic, and microwave the squash for about 15 minutes in an 800 watt microwave. Shorten the cooking time if you have a smaller squash or more powerful microwave. Let it sit in the bag in the microwave to steam, and then cool while you prepare the sauce. In a medium saucepan, combine a can of tomato sauce with the spices and sweetener. Let it simmer for a few minutes to allow the flavors to mix. Get a paper plate if you have one, or regular plate if you don't, and layer white (important to use plain white) paper napkins or paper towels on the plate. Put your pepperoni on the plate in a single layer, covering the plate. If you desire to cook up a lot, you can layer more towels/napkins and keep adding them to the same plate. Remove your spaghetti squash from the microwave. Put your pepperoni plate in and cook for 7-10 minutes. During that time you can slice your spaghetti squash open, remove the seeds and use a fork to put the strands in a bowl. Cover it with the sauce and mix well. Weigh out 8 oz. of the mixture and set aside, refrigerate the rest for another meal. Spray vegetable cooking spray over a ceramic ramekin or deep cereal bowl or small pyrex bowl and then put half of the spaghetti squash mixture in the bottom, mix the weighed cheeses cottage and soy cheeses) together and gently spread over the squash. Layer with the rest of the spaghetti squash mixture. Top with pepperoni. You can bake this in the oven at 350 degrees for 20 minutes, or if you want it finished quicker, you can nuke it for about 8 minutes and let sit to cool for a few. Reduce cheese to 1/2 ounce, if you can't find pure soy cheese. This recipe considers spaghetti squash to be summer squash; check with your sponsor first!

Ingredients

1/4 cup cottage cheese ◆ 1 ounce "mozarella" soy cheese and "parmesan" soy cheese mixed to your liking (combined weight) ◆ 1 ounce pepperoni, cooked briefly, as described below, then weighed ◆ 8 ounce cooked spaghetti squash with tomato sauce (combined weight) ◆ fresh or dried basil to taste ◆ 1 to 2 teaspoons garlic powder ◆ 1 to 2 teaspoons onion powder ◆ 1/2 teaspoon salt ◆ 1/2 to 1 teaspoon red pepper flakes ◆ 1/2 teaspoon oregano ◆ 1 to 2 packets of splenda/sweetener of your choice (but of course no sugar!)

Italian Sausage & Wild Mushrooms

Turn down to medium low and simmer until the juice is cooked down, stirring frequently(10-15 minutes.

Ingredients

3 lbs fresh wild mushrooms thinly sliced ◆ 1 lb hot italian sausage ◆ 1 28 oz can whole tomatoes; 3 cloves garlic ◆ 1/2 c olive oil ◆ 1/4 - 1/2 tsp crushed red pepper ◆ salt and pepper to taste

Jumbalaya

Before dicing, slice and salt eggplant and let it "bleed" for about an hour and rinse. Spray a skillet with PAM, add olive oil and heat. Put the sausage around the outside of pan. In the middle, drop the eggplant and onion. Cover and cook for about 30 minutes, stirring as needed. Add the tomatoes and sprinkle on Greek Seasoning. Cover and cook another 15 minutes or so. Salt and pepper to taste. Pan-fry.

Ingredients

1 1/2 cups diced eggplant ◆ 1/2 cup diced onion ◆ 1 cup diced tomato ◆ 1 teaspoon olive oil (optional) ◆ 4 oz sweet italian sausage ◆ greek seasoning

Kabocha Custard

To cook the squash, slice the top off around the stem as if you were carving a Jack O Lantern and remove gently, keeping it intact. Trim this section flat on the bottom. Scoop seeds out of squash. Add about 2 Tb water to the hollowed out squash, replace the top, and place on a dish in the microwave. Cook on high for 10-20 minutes, depending on the size of the squash and the strength of your microwave. (You can also place the squash in a saucepan on the stove. Add about 2 inches of water to the pan, cover, and steam. Be careful not to run out of water and burn the squash.) The skin of the squash will be tender to the touch when it is finished cooking. Slice open the squash and scoop the flesh into a large mixing bowl. Mash with fork, potato masher, or hand mixer. (Kabocha mashes quite easily, so the mixer is not required.) Measure out 4 or 8 oz (depending on how much winter squash you get) and set aside. If you are cooking this in a conventional oven, preheat to 350° F. For either microwave or conventional cooking, coat the inside of a 6-in diameter soufflé dish with the 1 Tb oil or butter. Whisk egg in large mixing bowl. Add milk and whisk thoroughly to blend. Whisk in sweetener, salt, and vanilla bean. Add the pre-measured squash and continue whisking until you have an even-textured, pale-yellow mixture. Pour this into the soufflé dish. If you are baking this in a conventional oven, place the soufflé dish in a baking tin with about ½ inch of water in it and bake for approximately one hour, until the top of the custard is firm. If you are using a microwave, cook on high power for about 20 minutes. The appearance of the finished custard should be fairly similar using either method, although the microwaved custard will pull away from the sides of the dish and the oven-baked version will not. Either way, the custard should be 'set' before you remove it from the oven. Measure portion and serve.

Ingredients

1 small kabocha squash ◆ 1 egg ◆ 1 cup milk ◆ sweetener ◆ salt ◆ dash ground vanilla bean ◆ 1 Tb light sweet oil such as coconut oil, almond oil, or walnut oil; or 1 Tb butter

Lox, Tomato, and Ricotta Cheese

Simply measure out some sliced tomatoes, sliced lox (smoked salmon), and ricotta cheese - you could also use some lettuce leaves - and either make little "sandwiches" or "rollups" with them. If you haven't guessed, the cheese replaces another kind of cheese we don't eat. (Labne can also be used in this recipe). Garnish with a little pepper or other spice.

Ingredients

Tomatoes ◆ Lox (smoked salmon) ◆ Ricotta Cheese

Mixed Grille for Indoor or Outdoor Grill

Start cooking zucchini and green peppers first, as they take the longest to cook. Remove from grill. Then cook tomatoes and onions. Remove from grill. Then cook protein. Weigh & measure for 16ozs vegetables and 4 ozs protein.

Ingredients

Zuchini ◆ green/red/yellow peppers ◆ onions tomatoes ◆ 5-6 ounces protein (chicken, salmon, shrimp, catfish, tilapia, chilean sea bass, london broil, lamb, steak, chicken livers, chops, hamburger, turkey burger, salmon burger, hard tofu)

Mixed Grille w/Vegetables & Protein

1. Weigh and measure about 20 oz vegetables. This will allow for about 4 oz water shrinkage in grilling and you can weigh and measure 16 oz (2 c) vegetables after cooking. 2. Weigh & measure about 5-6 oz protein: chicken, salmon, shrimp, catfish, tilapia, Chilean sea bass, London broil, lamb, steak, chicken livers, chops, hamburger, turkey burger, salmon burger, hard tofu. 3. Slice zucchini lengthwise. Slice green, red and yellow peppers into strips. Slice onions into quarters Slice tomatoes into 6ths. 4. Start cooking zucchini and green peppers first, as they take the longest to cook. Remove from grill. Then cook tomatoes and onions. Remove from grill. Then cook protein. 5. Weigh and measure for 16 oz vegetables and 4 oz protein.

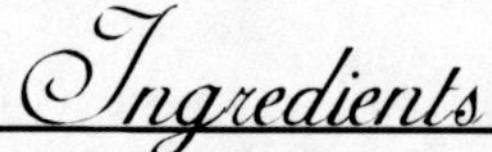

5-6 oz protein: chicken ◆ salmon ◆ shrimp ◆ catfish ◆ tilapia ◆ Chilean sea bass ◆ London broil ◆ lamb ◆ steak ◆ chicken livers ◆ chops ◆ hamburger ◆ turkey burger ◆ salmon burger ◆ hard tofu. ◆ Zucchini ◆ Green Peppers ◆ Red Peppers ◆ Yellow Peppers ◆ Onions ◆ Tomatoes

Mock Oat meal cookies

Mix ingredients together. Add water until mixture looks like cookie dough. Press on cookie sheet and bake at 350 degrees for approximately 20 minutes.

Ingredients

4 oz. TVP flakes ◆ 1/2 cup pumpkin ◆ salt ◆ cinnamon ◆ artificial sweetener to taste

Mushrooms and Mock "Barley"

Put just enough boiling water over the TVP for the water to be absorbed. Fry chopped onions and sliced mushrooms in olive oil Pam. Add butter, salt, and TVP to pan. When the butter melts, it's done.

Ingredients

1 oz. TVP ◆ 1/2 c onions and mushrooms ◆ 1 Tb Butter ◆ salt to taste

Mushrooms, Onions, and Soy

Cover texturized soy protein with boiling water until all liquid is absorbed. Spray skillet with zero-calorie butter spray. Cook onions and mushrooms in skillet, until onions are clear. Measure 1/2 cup. Add vegetables and measured portion of butter with texturized soy protein and mix.

Ingredients

1 ounce texturized soy protein ◆ 1/4 cup sauteed mushrooms ◆ 1/4 cup sauteed onions ◆ butter ◆ zero-calorie cooking spray ◆ salt

Pizza

Preheat oven to 400. Mix flour with enough water to make a moist dough. Make dough into ball and flatten into a pancake, nice and thin. Spray a baking dish liberally with Pam. Put the dough in the baking dish and sprinkle with salt, pepper, and garlic salt. Bake for about 20 minutes until golden brown. Spook tomato paste around the crust. Sprinkle with Italian Seasoning. Top with vegetables. Use a cheese grater and sprinkle cheese on top of vegetables. Put back into the oven until the cheese is melted and it looks done, maybe another 15 minutes or so.

Ingredients

2.5 oz soy flour ◆ 1.5 oz soy cheese–mozzarella style ◆ 2 tablespoons tomato paste ◆ 2 oz cooked onions ◆ 4 oz cooked peppers and mushrooms

Pork Chop w/Sauerkraut

Pan fry or broil 4 oz. pork chop. Heat or serve with 1 cup canned sauerkraut. Frying pan or broiler.

Ingredients

4 oz. pork chop ◆ 1 cup sauerkraut

Portobello Pizza

Slice off stem and carefully slice in half-like an English muffin so you have two circles from each mushroom. On microwaveable dish or tray, microwave the mushrooms only for about 2 to 3 minutes checking that they cook and shrink somewhat. Next, weigh out the mushroom (counts as cooked) and spread tomato paste on tops. Sprinkle garlic powder, add cheese, pepperoni and then oregano/basil. Microwave until cheese bubbles.

Ingredients

2 or 3 large portobello mushrooms ◆ 1/2 oz. tomato paste ◆ 1-1/2 oz. cheese or soy cheese ◆ 1/2 to 1 oz. pepperoni (optional) ◆ oregano ◆ basil ◆ garlic salt/powder

Pumpkin Cream Mock Souffle

Mix all ingredients in one bowl. Simmer on stove, or cook in microwave for several minutes. Great for Thanksgiving!

Ingredients

1/2 cup pumpkin ◆ 1 cup milk ◆ 1/2 teaspoon cinnamon ◆ 1/4 teaspoon ginger ◆ 1/4 teaspoon salt ◆ dash of clove ◆ sweetener

Pumpkin Custard

Mix pumpkin, sweetener, and spices in a bowl. Whisk in butter, egg, and milk. Pour into custard cups. Bake at 375° for approximately one hour. (Note: makes only 1/2 a cooked vegetable for those on maintenance.)

Ingredients

---

4 oz Canned Pumpkin ◆ 1/4 teaspoon Cinnamon ◆ 1/8 teaspoon Salt ◆ 1/8 teaspoon Ground Ginger ◆ 1/8 teaspoon Nutmeg ◆ 1/8 teaspoon Ground Cloves ◆ 1 Egg ◆ 1/4 cup Milk ◆ 1 teaspoon Butter melted ◆ 1 teaspoon Liquid Sweetener

Pumpkin Loaf

Preheat oven to 400° F. Beat the egg, water, spices, sweetener and salt together in a large bowl with a whisk. Add soy flour and beat until smooth. Fold in pumpkin (and wheat germ if you would normally have 8 oz pumpkin) with a large spatula. Pour the 1 tablespoon peanut (or other vegetable) oil into a small loaf pan and tilt the pan until the bottom is entirely coated with oil. Pour the pumpkin mixture into the pan. Bake for 30-40 minutes. Serve with 1 tablespoon butter or margarine.

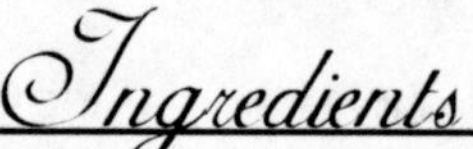

---

1 Egg ◆ 1/4 cup Water ◆ 1 teaspoon each Cinnamon ◆ Nutmeg ◆ Ginger ◆ Allspice ◆ 1 tablespoon Liquid Sweetener ◆ 1 teaspoon Salt ◆ 2 oz Soy Flour ◆ 4 oz Pumpkin, (2 tablespoon Wheat Germ) ◆ 1 tablespoon Peanut Oil ◆ 1 tablespoon Butter

Pumpkin Pie

Beat the egg, and mix all ingredients together. Put in microwave dish, sprayed with Pam, and cover loosely. Microwave approximately 3 minutes until set.

Ingredients

1 egg ◆ 1/2 cup pumpkin ◆ 3/4 teaspoon cinnamon ◆ 1/3 teaspoon ginger ◆ 1/4 teaspoon nutmeg, dash of ground cloves if desired ◆ sweetener

Pumpkin Tempeh Bread

Combine all ingredients and flatten like a tortilla on a cookie sheet that has been sprayed with non-stick spray. Bake at 350 for approximately 15 minutes.

Ingredients

1/2 cup canned pumpkin ◆ 3-½ oz. Tempeh ◆ 1/2 oz. Soy flour (Arrow Mills) ◆ 2 tablespoons Club soda ◆ 1/2 teaspoon Cinnamon, ◆ 1/4 teaspoon Celtic salt ◆ Sweeten to taste or 2 envelops artificial sweetener or Stevia

Pumpkin Yogurt Delight

Bring pumpkin to a boil in the microwave. Add allowable portion of butter, cinnamon, and sweetener; mix well. Add yogurt, stir thoroughly. Freeze for 2 hours.

Ingredients

1/2 cup yogurt ◆ 1/2 cup pumpkin ◆ butter ◆ 1/2 teaspoon cinnamon sweetener

Pumpkin Yummy

Stir together and nuke or bake until the cheese melts.

Ingredients

4 oz canned Pumpkin w/o sugar ◆ cinnamon and cloves (little bit) ◆ 1 tablespoon Roasted Sesame Oil ◆ 1 Egg ◆ 1 oz Wheat Germ ◆ 1 oz Soy Cheddar Cheese ◆ 1 oz Soy Nuts

Quiche Recipe

Spray the bottom of a small Tupperware container with Pam. Mix the grated cheese and veggie together and press into the bottom of the dish. Beat the egg whites with 2 tablespoons of water, salt, pepper and a bit of nutmeg. Pour the whites over the cheese and vegetables and microwave until set (about 3 or 4 minutes).

Ingredients

2 oz. egg whites ◆ 1 oz. grated cheese ◆ 4 oz. cooked chopped vegetable ◆ salt ◆ pepper ◆ nutmeg to taste

Rita's Hawaiian Spaghetti Squash Dinner (or Lunch)

Toss squash with butter, cinnamon and sweetener. Top with ham and soy nuts.

Ingredients

8 oz. cooked spaghetti squash ◆ 1 tablespoon butter or margarine ◆ 1/2 teaspoon cinnamon (more or less to taste) ◆ 1 packet sweetener 3 oz. cooked ◆ diced ham ◆ 1 oz. soy nuts

Rita's Um-m-m! Chicken Salad

Melt butter in a small skillet. Add onion, diced chicken, and soy sauce; toss until warm. Mix dressing and salsa together. Add bacon, salsa/dressing mixture, and finally chicken and onion to salad.

Ingredients

1 Grey Sheet dinner salad with no dressing ◆ 4 oz. combination diced ◆ cooked chicken breast and cooked bacon ◆ 3 oz. onion (cooked in microwave 8 minutes) ◆ 1 oz. salsa, hot or mild ◆ 2 Tb Ranch dressing ◆ 1 Tb soy sauce ◆ 1 Tb butter or margarine

Salad, Taco Style

Measure out taco-style salad vegetables, such as lettuce, tomato, carrots, etc. Stir cooked ground beef or soy in with cooked onions and tomato sauce. Top salad with cooked meat and onions. Add allowable portion of ranch dressing on top.

Ingredients

2 cups salad ◆ 4 ounces cooked ground beef or 4 ounces cooked ground soy, such as Gimme Lean ◆ 1/2 cup sauteed onions ◆ 2 ounces tomato sauce, taco spices or abstinent seasoned salt, ranch dressing

Sallie's Pumpkin Pie

Combine the soy flour with the butter and salt to form a single pie crust. Bake the completed pie shell at 350°F for 10 minutes. Beat the egg, spices, sweetener, and salt in a large bowl. Add pumpkin and 1/8-1/4 cup water and beat until smooth. The mixture should be about the consistency of pancake batter: thick but liquid. Pour pumpkin mixture into crust and bake for 20-30 minutes. Pie is done when a fork stuck into the middle comes out clean.

Ingredients

2 oz Soy Flour ◆ 1 tablespoons Butter ◆ 1 teaspoon Salt ◆ 4 Oz Pumpkin ◆ 1 Egg ◆ 1 teaspoon Cinnamon ◆ 1/2 teaspoon Ginger ◆ 1/4 teaspoon Cloves ◆ 1 tablespoon Liquid Sweetener ◆ 1/2 teaspoon Salt

Sauerkraut and Bacon, Fried

Melt allowable portion of margarine in frying pan. Add drained sauerkraut. Sprinkle with salt and pepper. Saute until browned. Add bacon or frankfurters and serve.

Ingredients

4 ounces bacon or cut up frankfurters ◆ 8 ounces sauerkraut drained ◆ salt and pepper ◆ margarine

Sauteed Chicken with Portobello Mushrooms & Red Bell Peppers

Saute peppers and mushrooms in olive oil or butter. After cooked, measure out 1 c. vegetable and set aside. Continue to quick saute 4 ozs chicken breast on high heat. Reduce heat and cover. Cook 20 minutes. In last 2 minutes re-add previously cooked vegetables.

Ingredients

1 cup red bell peppers ◆ 1 c portobello mushrooms ◆ 1 tbs olive oil or butter ◆ 4 oz. Chicken breast

Shag Panir (Indian Spinach, Tomatoes and Cheese)

Combine spinach with chopped or crushed tomatoes - either even quantities, or use more spinach than tomatoes. Sautee in butter, adding in Indian spices. (Spices are to taste. You can use either a prepared curry powder, or a garam masala, or a mixture of cumin, turmeric, coriander, red pepper, and anything else you like). After the vegetables are cooked and measured, add your measured ricotta cheese, and, if desired, some tomato sauce or paste (optional), and sweetener to taste (also optional). If the vegetables are hot enough, it will not be necessary to reheat after adding the ricotta, but you may wish too.

Ingredients

Spinach (either fresh, canned, or frozen and thawed) ◆ chopped or crushed Tomatoes ◆ Butter (peanut oil works too) ◆ Indian spices

Sherry's Pumpkin Delight

Bring pumpkin to a boil in microwave. Add butter, cinnamon, and sweetener; mix well. Add yogurt, stir thoroughly. Freeze for 2 hours.

Ingredients

4 oz. canned pumpkin ◆ 1/2 cup yogurt ◆ 1 tablespoon butter ◆ 1/2 teaspoon cinnamon ◆ 1 package sweetener

Shrimp and Cabbage Salad

Combine celery, cabbage, and tomatoes. Stir in mustard and allowable portion of mayonnaise. Chill for 2 to 3 hours. Add shrimp, salt, and pepper, and serve.

Ingredients

4 oz. cooked ◆ chilled shrimp ◆ 1 cup chopped shredded cabbage ◆ 1/2 cup chopped celery ◆ 1/2 cup sliced tomatoes ◆ 1 tablespoon mustard ◆ mayonnaise ◆ salt and pepper

Soy Bean Dip

Mix everything in a food processor or blender until smooth. When weighing the tomatoes and mushrooms, you may wish to include some of the juices from the tomatoes in your measurement to help the consistency of the dip. Pour the processed or blended mixture into a microwaveable container and heat on high for about 3 minutes (more if your microwave is lower wattage). You can use that time to clean and ready your raw veggies. *Can be fresh (raw) but you should increase your cooking time accordingly.

Ingredients

3 ounces canned soy beans* ◆ 1 ounce grated or shredded soy cheese ◆ 8 ounces canned chopped tomatoes with green chiles (sometimes sold by the brand name RoTel) and drained ◆ canned mushrooms* ◆ 1/4 to 1/2 teaspoon hot red pepper flakes ◆ 1/2 teaspoon garlic powder ◆ 1 teaspoon onion powder ◆ 1/2 teaspoon ground celery seed (celery powder) ◆ 1/2 teaspoon salt (or to taste), ◆ Raw veggies from Lunch Finger Salad or Dinner Salad

Soy Crust Spinach Pizza

Combine crust ingredients and flatten like a tortilla on a cookie sheet that has been sprayed with non-stick spray. Bake at 350 degrees for approximately 15 minutes. Remove crust from oven and put on the topping. Return to oven and cook until cheese is melted.

Ingredients

3 oz. soy flour ◆ ¼ to ½ cup Club soda ◆ ¼ teaspoon Celtic salt. ◆ ¼ cup cooked onions ◆ ½ cup spinach ◆ ¼ cup pizza sauce ◆ 1 oz. soy mozzarella cheese ◆ ¼ teaspoon Celtic salt

Soy Pizza

Weigh soy flour. Add enough water to soy flour to make a ball. Spray hands liberally with zero-calorie butter spray. Shape soy flour into ball, and then spread out as thin as possible. Pan fry in pan liberally coated in zero-calorie butter spray. Microwave pepperoni in paper towels. Sauté mushrooms in zero-calorie butter spray and garlic. Weigh and measure cooked pepperoni and mushrooms. Layer all on cooked soy flour and serve. Serving Variations: Use 1 oz. soy cheese by reducing soy flour and pepperoni to 1 1/2 oz. each. Use 3/4 cup mushrooms and 1/4 cup chopped tomatoes with green chiles (RoTel). Use 1 cup artichoke hearts and 1 oz. Roquefort cheese instead of mushrooms and pepperoni. Season soy flour with abstinent spices or allowable portion of juice from canned tomatoes or jalapeno peppers.

Ingredients

2 ounces soy flour or finely ground texturized soy protein ◆ 2 ounces pepperoni ◆ 1 cup mushrooms ◆ zero-calorie butter spray ◆ garlic

Soy Pizza, Large Crust

Preheat oven to 550° F or as hot as it will go. Heat the pizza stone or baking sheet inside the oven. Mix texturized soy protein, garlic powder, salt, oil, and cold water to form a firm ball of dough (use a fork). Add the water a little at a time to avoid making an unusable mess. Roll between sheets of non-stick baking paper until you have a flat pizza about 1/2 inch thick. Place dough on the preheated pizza stone or pizza pan. Bake for 5 minutes, until dry and somewhat golden. Remove from oven, spread the vegetables and tomato sauce, and bake for another 8 minutes.

Ingredients

4 ounces finely ground texturized soy protein ◆ 1 teaspoon garlic powder ◆ salt ◆ 1 tablespoon sesame oil (fat from salad) or 2 teaspoon zero calorie butter spray, approx ◆ 1/4 cup water ◆ 1 cup cooked vegetables, such as zucchini, mushrooms, tomatoes with Italian seasonings ◆ 2 ounces tomato sauce

Soyloaf

Mix ingredients together. Pour it into a large sprayed loaf pan and bake at 350 degrees for about 45 minutes.

Ingredients

2 oz. soy flour ◆ 1 egg ◆ 1 oz. flavoring ◆ 8 oz. flavor seltzer ◆ 1 oz. wheatgerm ◆ 16 oz. cooked vegetable (use your favorite ones) ◆ spices

Spaghetti Squash alla Gorgonzola

Pierce several holes in spaghetti squash with a paring knife. Microwave approximately 15 minutes, rotating a quarter turn every 4 or 5 minutes. (Squash is done when tender but not mushy to the touch.) Slice squash open, remove seeds, and loosen strands with a fork. Weigh 8 oz. of the cooked squash, add remaining ingredients, and microwave until cheese and butter are melted (about 2 minutes).

Ingredients

1 spaghetti squash ◆ 1 1/2 oz. gorgonzola or bleu cheese ◆ 1/2 oz parmesan or Romano cheese ◆ 1 tablespoon butter ◆ salt and pepper

Spinach Pizza with Soy Crust

Combine all the above ingredients and flatten like a tortilla on a cookie sheet that has been sprayed with non-stick spray. Bake at 350 for approximately 15 minutes. Remove crust from oven and put on the topping. Return to oven and cook till cheese is melted.

Ingredients

Crust: 3 oz. Soy flour (Arrow Mills) ◆ ¼ to ½ cup Club soda (till it makes dough. You will have to keep hands wet in order for the dough not to stick to them when you are patting it flat) ◆ ¼ tsp. Celtic salt (or salt to taste) ◆ ¼ cup cooked onions ◆ ½ cup spinach ◆ ¼ cup pizza sauce (check ingredients or just make your own from tomato sauce) ◆ 1 oz. Soy Mozzarella cheese ◆ ¼ tsp. Celtic salt

The Faithful Tried & True Omelet

Microwave 3 minutes or cook in a pan until done.

Ingredients

2 Eggs ◆ 1/2 cup carrots ◆ 1 cup chopped tomato, green beans, celery, cabbage, onion, green pepper (however you like it) ◆ 1 tablespoon Oil

Tofu with Broccoli Stirfry

Heat skillet or wok until very hot. Stirfry the broccoli fast and hot. Cover the skillet or wok and steam the broccoli for a few minutes.Add the mushrooms and tofu and stirfry quickly until hot.

Ingredients

2 Eggs ◆ 1/2 cup carrots ◆ 1 cup chopped tomato, green beans, celery, cabbage, onion, green pepper (however you like it) ◆ 1 tablespoon Oil

Tuna Melty

Broil in toaster oven or cook in oven until the cheese gets toasted on top (roughly 5 minutes)

Ingredients

1 oz. raw wheat germ ◆ 2 oz. Tuna ◆ 1 oz. sliced cheese (swiss or muenster are good) ◆ 1 plum tomato (or part of large tomato), 1 tbs. mayonnaise

Wheat Germ and Goat Cheese

Dice cheese and mix with wheat germ and oil. Microwave 30 seconds at a time on defrost, being careful not to burn the cheese. Stir with edge of knife. Good warm or cold.

Ingredients

2 Tb wheat germ (4 Tb for maintenance) ◆ 1 Tb peanut oil ◆ 2 oz. Gjetost goat cheese

Zucchini Soy Nut Butter Flatbread

Mix all ingredients thoroughly and spread into one of those oddly shaped foil soufflé pans you get in most grocery stores...try the cooking gadgets department. Bake for 30 minutes, longer if you wish a crunchier treat.

Ingredients

1 Egg ◆ 3/4 oz Soy Flour ◆ 1 1/4 oz Soy Nut Butter ◆ 3/4 oz Wheat Germ ◆ 2 oz Finely chopped (then steamed) Zucchini ◆ Stevia for sweetening ◆ Frontier Flavors of choice

Chicken with Spinach, Garlic, and Tomato Sauce

Grill chicken breasts for 5 minutes on each side, until cooked through but not dry. Meanwhile, lightly brown the garlic in a nonstick skillet, sprayed with zero-calorie butter spray, over medium-high heat. Add the spinach and cook, tossing gently, just until leaves are wilted. Add the tomatoes, soy sauce, and vinegar. Toss well until coated and thoroughly heated. Weigh 4 ounces of chicken. Measure 1 cup of spinach and tomatoes. Place spinach and tomatoes on top of cooked chicken, and serve.

Ingredients

4 boneless skinless chicken breast halves (about 2 pounds total) ◆ 6 cups washed loosely packed spinach (about 1 1/2 pounds) ◆ 1 cup plum tomatoes ◆ 8-12 cloves garlic, minced ◆ 2 teaspoons soy sauce ◆ 1/4 cup vinegar ◆ zero-calorie butter spray

Lobster and Cauliflower Salad

Marinate the cauliflower in vinegar for 2 hours. Drain. Combine with lobster and toss with allowable portion of mayonnaise and mustard. Variations: 4 oz. shrimp, or 2 oz. lobster and 1 hard boiled egg, sliced.

Ingredients

4 ounces cooked lobster chunks ◆ 2 cups cauliflower, washed and cut into paper-thin slices ◆ mustard ◆ mayonnaise ◆ vinegar

Souvlakia

For the vegetables, combine marinade ingredients with about 1 cup water in a large saucepan and bring to a boil. Drop in mushrooms and stir to coat, about 1 minute. Drop in onions and green pepper, ditto. Remove pan from heat and let stand uncovered until cool. Add tomatoes and stir thoroughly. Transfer to a large container, cover, and marinate overnight in the refrigerator. For the meat, combine marinade ingredients in a large container. Add the meat and stir to coat thoroughly. Marinate in the refrigerator overnight. When the meat and vegetables have been thoroughly marinated, either thread them onto skewers and barbecue them or broil them in the oven.

Ingredients

Meat: 2 lbs lamb or beef cut into large chunks ◆ 2 large yellow onions peeled and cut into quarters ◆ 2 large green bell peppers cut into 1 1/2-inch chunks ◆ 1 lb fresh white mushrooms cleaned ◆ 6 plum or cherry tomatoes ◆ left whole, Marinade (make 1 for meat, 1 for vegetables) ◆ 3 Tb good olive oil ◆ 2 Tb balsamic vinegar ◆ 1 Tb lemon juice ◆ 3 cloves garlic pressed ◆ 2 bay leaves crumbled ◆ 2 Tb fresh or dried basil ◆ 2 Tb dried oregano ◆ pinch thyme ◆ pinch crushed rosemary ◆ salt and pepper to taste

Spinach-Artichoke Dip

Heat oven to 350°F. Spray an ovenproof pan with Pam or zero-calorie butter spray. In a food processor, process spinach, artichokes, garlic, ricotta cheese, Parmesan, and pepper until well combined, scraping down sides of processor, as needed. Spread mixture in prepared pan.

Ingredients

3 ounces ricotta cheese ◆ 1/2 ounce grated Parmesan cheese ◆ 1/2 cup frozen chopped spinach ◆ thawed ◆ 1/2 cup artichoke bottoms ◆ 2 cloves garlic ◆ 1/4 teaspoon freshly ground pepper

Texturized Soy Protein Thai Salad

Combine texturized soy protein with 1/2 cup hot water and unsweetened ketchup. Let stand 5 minutes. Meanwhile, combine soy sauce, vinegar, garlic, red pepper, sweetener, and lemon juice, and set aside. Slice carrots and green onion. Shred cabbage. Combine soy protein mixture with soy sauce mixture in a microwaveable dish. Cover with plastic wrap and microwave on medium-high for 8 minutes, until chunks are tender and liquid is absorbed. Heat a large non-stick skillet or wok sprayed with zero-calorie butter spray. Stir-fry the soy protein for about 3-5 minutes until browned. Add salad veggies to wok and spray them with Pam. Mix with soy protein for about 1 minute or less until they are lightly warmed but still raw. Remove and top with sesame oil, for dressing.

Ingredients

4 ounces chunk style texturized soy protein (these are larger chunks of soy granules, about 1/4 cubed, if you can find them) ◆ 2 cups salad - thinly sliced carrots and regular, or Chinese, cabbage, and green onions, if desired ◆ 1 ounce unsweetened ketchup or tomato sauce with spices ◆ 1 ounce soy sauce, 3 tablespoons vinegar ◆ 1 teaspoon garlic, minced ◆ sweetener ◆ 1/8 - 1/2 teaspoon red pepper ◆ 1 tablespoon lemon juice ◆ 1 tablespoons sesame oil (fat) ◆ zero-calorie butter spray

Tofu Cacciatore

To squeeze excess moisture from tofu, place tofu slices on a baking sheet. Cover with parchment paper or plastic wrap and set a second baking sheet on top. Place weights (heavy cans or pans) on top of the baking sheet. Set aside for 15 minutes. (Or, if you want a meatier texture, spread tofu slices on a baking sheet, cover with plastic wrap and freeze until ready to use.) Preheat oven to 350 degrees F (175 degrees C). Spray a saute pan once with cooking spray and place pan over low heat. Add peppers and cook, stirring frequently, for 5 minutes. Add garlic, basil, and oregano and cook, stirring, for 15 seconds. Stir in tomatoes and tomato paste. Cover and simmer for 15 minutes. While sauce is simmering, spray a large saute pan or griddle once with cooking spray and place pan over low heat. Brown the tofu in the pan lightly on both sides. Measure 4 ounces tofu and 8 ounces cooked vegetables. Individual servings can be placed in pyrex baking cups. Cover tofu with tomato-pepper sauce. Cover baking cups with parchment paper and aluminum foil. Bake for 30 - 45 minutes -- the longer they bake, the more flavor the tofu will absorb. Variations: 1 medium onion may be added with peppers on maintenance. If allowed, use 1/2 portion of cooked vegetable to stir-fry tofu in wheat germ, and use other 1/2 portion cooked vegetable to cover tofu with tomato-pepper sauce.

Ingredients

2 pounds firm tofu, cut into 1/2 inch thick slices ◆ 2 bell peppers, cored and sliced ◆ 3 5-ounce cans chopped tomatoes, drained ◆ 2 tablespoons tomato paste ◆ 1 tablespoon finely chopped fresh garlic ◆ 2 teaspoons dried basil ◆ 2 teaspoons dried oregano ◆ zero-calorie butter spray ◆ salt ◆ pepper

Tomato, Baked

Preheat oven to 350F and spray a baking pan with cooking spray. Place the tomatoes cut side up on the pan and sprinkle evenly with the black pepper, garlic powder, parmesan and then the oregano. Bake until the tomatoes are tender but not squishy. Approximately 8 - 12 minutes depending on the size and ripeness of the tomatoes. Measure 1 cup tomatoes and top with 1 ounce parmesan cheese. Microwave with cheese, if desired.

Ingredients

1/2 ounce parmesan cheese ◆ 2 large ripe but firm tomatoes, cut in half ◆ 1 teaspoon oregano ◆ 1/4 teaspoon fresh ground black pepper ◆ 1/2 teaspoon garlic powder ◆ zero-calorie cooking spray

Tongue and Spinach Salad

Toss the tongue, bacon, spinach, and horseradish with allowable portion of vinaigrette dressing.

Ingredients

3 1/2 ounces julienne of tongue ◆ 1/2 ounce bacon bits ◆ 2 cups spinach leaves ◆ 1 tablespoon horseradish ◆ vinaigrette dressing

Tuna Salad

Flake the tuna. Combine with celery and onion. Bind with allowable portion of mayonnaise. Serve on greens.

Ingredients

1/2 cup white-meat tuna ◆ 1 cup finely cut celery ◆ 3/4 cup greens ◆ 1/4 cup finely chopped onion ◆ 1/2 teaspoon salt ◆ 1/2 teaspoon pepper ◆ mayonnaise

Winter Squash, Spaghetti a la Gorgonzola

Split spaghetti squash lengthwise and remove seeds. Place flat side of squash down in a microwave dish with about ½ inch water and cover. Cook on high for approximately 15-30 minutes. (Squash is done when tender but not mushy to the touch.) Loosen strands with a fork. Measure out 1/2 cup of the cooked squash. Add remaining ingredients, and microwave until cheese and butter are melted (about 2 minutes). Top with additional zero calorie butter spray, if desired.

Ingredients

1 whole spaghetti winter squash ◆ 1 1/2 ounces gorgonzola or bleu cheese ◆ 1/2 ounce Parmesan or Romano cheese ◆ butter ◆ salt, and pepper

Winter Squash, Spaghetti Hawaiian Style

Toss squash with butter, cinnamon, and sweetener. Top with ham and soy nuts. Add additional zero calorie butter spray, if desired.

Ingredients

3 ounces cooked, diced ham ◆ 1 ounce soy nuts ◆ 1/2 cup spaghetti winter squash, butter or margarine ◆ 1/2 teaspoon cinnamon (more or less, to taste) ◆ sweetener

Yellow Squash Frittata

Boil squash until tender; drain and chop up quite small. Measure 1 cup of squash and set aside. Beat egg with the grated cheese, Italian seasoning, salt and pepper. Spray frying pan with zero-calorie butter spray, and add 1 cup squash. Pour egg mixture over squash. Cook until egg is cooked and puffy. Variation: Use only 1/2 cup cooked squash for this recipe and use 1/2 portion cooked vegetable for something else. Use 2 eggs and no cheese, if preferred.

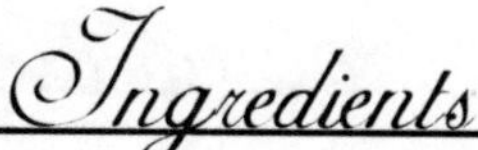

2 - 3 yellow summer squash ◆ 1 egg ◆ 1 ounce cheese, grated ◆ Italian seasoning ◆ zero-calorie butter spray ◆ salt and pepper

Zucchini Broiled with Parmesan Cheese

Heat broiler. Place rack 4-inches from heating element. Leaving stem ends attached, cut zucchini lengthwise into 1/4" slices. Place on a baking sheet and carefully fan out slices. Spray with zero-calorie butter spray. Sprinkle with salt and pepper. Broil about 6 minutes or until zucchini is softened. Carefully spread fans out more. Sprinkle with cheese. Broil 5 to 6 minutes more, until cheese is lightly browned.

Ingredients

2 ounces grated Parmesan cheese ◆ 1 cup zucchini summer squash, thinly sliced longways, in fan shapes ◆ zero-calorie butter spray (olive oil flavored) ◆ 1/2 teaspoon salt ◆ 1/4 teaspoon pepper

Gingersnap Cookie

Mash dry ingredients in bowl, add small amount water, keeping it dry and able to pack well. Cook 60 seconds in microwave egg/muffin cup. Let cool. Very good for traveling.

Ingredients

Wheat Germ (your legal measurement) ◆ Small amt liquid, (water, diet soda) ◆ Sweetener ◆ Powdered ginger (spice)

Wheat Germ Vegetable

GS Cookies

First spray the microwave dish with buttered flavored spray. Bake in microwave for a few minutes. You'll have to judge how long to bake. My microwave cooks slow so I watch it. I'll bake it for about 2-3 minutes. Then more if needed. You can bake it soft or tougher.

Ingredients

1 oz. Wheat Germ ◆ Flavoring to taste
◆ Diet Soda/flavored club soda or seltzer

Wheat Germ Cupcakes

1. In a separate container (a Rubbermaid cup works well) mix the wheat germ with a few abundant shakes of ground cinnamon, ground ginger (less than cinnamon), and black pepper (less than ginger) and add the optional sesame seeds (some people use poppy seeds). If you don't like sweet or spicy food, try something else - like garlic salt and perhaps mild mustard seeds. 2. Melt the butter in about 1/2 cup of hot tap water (1/4 cup if you're on 1/8 cup wheat germ) and add liquid sweetener to taste [I used Sweet & Low and Cyclamate (the latter not available in the US)]. (Don't know if powdered would work - maybe Stevia?) This is where you'd be able alternatively to use, e.g., garlic salt and mustard seeds. 3. Stir the liquid into the dry mixture. 4. Spray the baking tin with butter-flavored Pam or a similar product. 5. Spoon the mixture into the baking receptacle. (doesn't have to be cupcake tins.) My preference is to bake it for a long time on low heat so it resembles what they used to give babies when they're teething! Since there's nothing in the ingredients that NEEDS cooking, the heat is just to make it firm enough to pick up. This recipe was given me by a long-term abstinent Cambridge Greysheeter gourmet. It could be made without sweetener - the basic thing to know is that the combination of wheat germ, water, and fat can be baked into a stable, crunchy (or soft, if you prefer) Grey Sheet food portion.

Ingredients

1 oz wheat germ (If you're on 1/8 cup wheat germ, halve the recipe) ◆ 1 1/2 teaspoon butter or margarine ◆ 1/2 cup water ◆ 1 tablespoon sesame seeds (check with sponsor) ◆ sweetener and/or spice if desired

Wheatgerm cookies

Mix well. Spray small round microwave container with non stick cooking spray. Microwave 6 minutes. Let cool or freeze. Eat with margarine.

Ingredients

1 oz. wheat germ ◆ 3 tablespoons cinnamon ◆ 2 Equals ◆ 1/2 teaspoon orange rind ◆ 3 oz. cream soda

Fake sandwich

Cook in hot sandwich maker for 5 to 10 minutes (pre-sprayed with Mazola 0 calorie butter spray). When cooled down or warm, cut bread in half and spread soynut butter.

Ingredients

1 oz. wheatgerm ◆ 1 egg ◆ 1 tablespoon banana flavoring and maple flavoring ◆ pinch of salt ◆ 2 oz. soynut butter ◆ 2 tablespoons soda water to fluff

Muesli

Mix and serve.

Ingredients

1/2 cup yogurt ◆ 2 ounces soy nuts ◆ 1/8 cup wheat germ ◆ 1 1/2 teaspoon peanut, walnut, or hazelnut oil (optional from fat measurement) or abstinent extract, to taste (vanilla, chocolate, almond)

Soy butter travel bars

Beat all the ingredients together. Bake at 350 degrees for about 30 to 35 minutes.

Ingredients

1 egg ◆ 1 oz. yogurt ◆ 2 tablespoons wheat germ ◆ 1 1/2 teaspoon butter or oil ◆ 1/2 teaspoon salt ◆ 1 teaspoon cinnamon (you also could use powdered vanilla bean, or extracts) ◆ 2 to 3 tablespoons Equal, water

Spinach Quiche

Beat egg in a straight-sided plastic container. Add wheat germ, salt, pepper, and spices of your choice. Add spinach and cheese. Top with allowable portion of butter. Microwave about 4 minutes. Makes a good travel food, and tastes good hot or cold!

Ingredients

1 egg ◆ 1 ounce feta cheese ◆ 1 tablespoon wheat germ ◆ 1/2 cup cooked spinach ◆ salt ◆ pepper ◆ spices ◆ butter

Raw Vegetable

Broccoli Salad

Mix together.

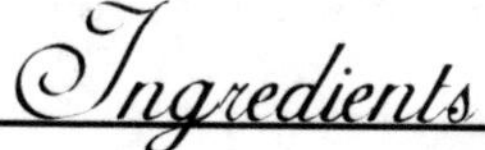

chopped raw broccoli ◆ chopped celery ◆ 1 oz. mixed soy nuts and bacon bits ◆ 1 tablespoon mayonnaise

Cabbage and Carrot Cole Slaw

Measure cabbage and carrots into one bowl. Add allowable portion of mayonnaise and vinegar and mix together. Prepare a few minutes early, and let the mixture sit, to fully marry the flavors together.Restir and serve. For a sweeter cole slaw, add more sweetener.

Ingredients

2 cups shredded cabbage and carrots ◆ mayonnaise ◆ vinegar to taste ◆ salt and pepper, or abstinent seasoned salt ◆ sweetener

Cabbage and Pepper Fiesta Slaw

Slice red and white cabbage in a food processor, or grater, or by hand, in long thin strips. Dice red, green, and yellow bell peppers into small cubes. Toss together. After measuring one serving, measure your oil allowance, and add on top. You may also add a few drops of lemon juice.

Ingredients

Red cabbage ◆ White cabbage ◆ Red bell pepper ◆ Green bell pepper ◆ Yellow bell pepper

Carrot Salad

Peel carrots and either food process or grate by hand to make a shredded slaw consistency. Mix in mayo, sweetener to taste, and just a dash of salt. Food Processor. Refrigerate

Ingredients

3 raw carrots ◆ 1 teaspoon mayonnaise ◆ sweetener to taste ◆ dash salt

Chicken Salad

Melt allowable portion of margarine in a small skillet. Add onion, diced chicken, and soy sauce; toss until warm. Mix allowable portion of salad dressing and ketchup together. Add bacon, salsa/dressing mixture, and finally chicken and onion to salad.

Ingredients

4 ounces combination diced, cooked chicken breast and cooked bacon ◆ 1/2 cup onion (cooked in microwave 8 minutes) ◆ 2 cups salad ranch dressing ◆ 1 tablespoon soy sauce ◆ 2 tablespoons diet ketchup with onion and chili powder to taste ◆ margarine

Claussen Crunch

Mix the cauliflower, tomatoes, dill pickles, onion and dill weed in a large bowl, then transferred it to a gallon zip-lock bag. Then I measured out 8 ounces of this mixture, and since I was having it for lunch today, I added 1 tablespoon of Ranch Dressing. I let this mixture set overnight in a covered Tupperware container in the fridge, then this morning, I added 1 ounce of the black soybeans, and mixed well.

Ingredients

1 head Cauliflower rinsed, trimmed, cut in bite-size pieces ◆ 15-20 Cherry Tomatoes cut in 1/4ths (or 2 large tomatoes, chopped) ◆ 4-5 Kosher Dill Pickle Spears cut in 1/2" slices ◆ 1/2 small Onion peeled & chopped ◆ 1 teaspoon Dill Weed ◆ 1 oz. White or Black canned Soy Beans ◆ 1 tablespoons Ranch Dressing (depending on which meal you are eating it at) ◆ Salt & Pepper to taste

Club Salad

Stir allowable portion of mayonnaise into chicken. Place lettuce leaves on plate. Add tomatoes. Add chicken. Top with bacon.

Ingredients

3 1/2 ounces chicken ◆ 1/2 ounce bacon ◆ 1 1/2 cups lettuce ◆ 1/2 cup diced tomatoes, ◆ mayonnaise

Cole Slaw

Shred cabbage finely. Crisp cabbage in cold water for an hour. Drain well. Measure portion for salad serving. Add allowable portion of mayonnaise and seasonings. Toss well and let stand for 30 minutes or longer. Serve cold.

Ingredients

1 head cabbage ◆ mayonnaise ◆ 1 teaspoon Dijon mustard ◆ salt ◆ pepper

Crab Louis

Mix crab, tomato sauce, and allowable portion of mayonnaise together. Serve on top of 2 cups lettuce. This is best made with Dungeness crab, but lump crabmeat is almost as good. Meat from lobster tails may also be used. Variation: 1/4 cup crab and 1 hard-boiled egg, sliced.

Ingredients

1/2 cup crab ◆ 2 cups shredded lettuce ◆ 2 ounces tomato sauce or chili sauce ◆ mayonnaise

Crab Salad

Mix greens, celery, and onion. Stir in mustard and allowable portion of mayonnaise. Chill for 2 to 3 hours. Top with crabmeat and serve.

Ingredients

1/2 cup crabmeat ◆ 1 1/4 cup lettuce greens ◆ 1/2 cup finely cut celery ◆ 1/4 cup finely cut onion ◆ mustard ◆ mayonnaise

Cucumbers and Cream

Whip cottage cheese, herbs, and salt to taste, in blender. Spread on cucumbers.

Ingredients

1/2 cup cottage cheese ◆ 3 raw, sliced cucumbers ◆ 2 teaspoons of fresh herbs (dill or chives) ◆ salt

Cucumbers, Dill

Save juice from dill pickles. Put cucumbers in jar with juice. Measure for raw veggies.

Ingredients

dill pickle juice ◆ cucumbers

Cucumbers, Sweet

Mix white vinegar and sweetener together. Pour mixture over cucumbers and green onions. Chill and add these to salad.

Ingredients

sliced cucumbers chopped green onions white vinegar sweetener

Egg Salad

Chop eggs roughly, or push them through the large-holed side of a four sided box grater. In a mixing bowl, mix eggs with allowable portion of mayonnaise, mustard, salt, and pepper into with a wooden spoon. Stir in chopped celery and tomato.

Ingredients

2 hardboiled eggs ◆ 2 cups chopped tomatoes and celery ◆ mayonnaise ◆ 1 tablespoon Dijon mustard ◆ 1/2 teaspoon salt, ◆ 1/4 teaspoon pepper

Fiesta Slaw

Slice red and white cabbage in a food processer or grater or by hand in long thin strips. Dice red and green and yellow bell pepper into small cubes. Toss together. Measure 1 c. or 8 ozs. Measure 1 tbs oil and add a few drips of lemon juice. Toss on Fiesta Slaw.

Ingredients

Red cabbage ◆ White cabbage ◆ Red bell pepper ◆ Green bell pepper ◆ Yellow bell pepper

Kimchee (Thai Cabbage)

Salt the cabbage and toss. Place in colander. Place weights on top. I do this in the morning and then later in the afternoon I do the rest. Take the cabbage add red pepper flakes, finely chopped fresh ginger, sweetener and rice vinegar. Depending on how hot and spicy you like your food that is how much of the red pepper flakes and ginger you should add.

Ingredients

Cabbage ◆ Red Pepper Flakes ◆ Ginger-fresh & chopped ◆ 2 packages Sweetener ◆ 1/4-1/2 cup Rice Vinegar

Lobster and Cauliflower Salad

Marinate the cauliflower in vinegar for 2 hours. Drain. Combine with lobster and toss with allowable portion of mayonnaise and mustard. Variations: 4 oz. shrimp, or 2 oz. lobster and 1 hard boiled egg, sliced.

Ingredients

4 ounces cooked lobster chunks ◆ 2 cups cauliflower, washed and cut into paper-thin slices ◆ mustard ◆ mayonnaise ◆ vinegar

Mock "Potato" Salad

Mix it all together and you've got potato salad. This is a good one to take to the office if you have a frig there. It makes a great side dish.Also, If you opt to make the squash softer by cooking longer, this recipe easily becomes a mock egg salad.

Ingredients

Butternut squash ◆ dill pickles ◆ chopped ◆ sweet onions ◆ chopped ◆ kerbie cucumbers ◆ raw carrots, cut up into small pieces and or red cabbage ◆ juice from dill pickles ◆ seasonings of your preference, including hot sauce ◆ dill, etc.

Mushroom and Bibb Lettuce Salad

Wash Bibb lettuce thoroughly. Place the Bibb and mushrooms in a bowl. Sprinkle with parsley. Measure 2 cups and allowable portion of vinaigrette dressing Bibb comes in small heads, is exceptionally green and crisp, and maintains its crispness extremely well in a salad. It is, however, difficult to clean and requires thorough rinsing and soaking. Tear off the leaves, or break the heads into quarters or halves, according to size.

Ingredients

4 to 6 heads Bibb lettuce, cut in quarters ◆ 1/2 pound white mushrooms, stemmed and thinly sliced ◆ 2 tablespoons chopped parsley ◆ vinaigrette dressing

No Mayo Cole Slaw

Mix together

Ingredients

1 package pre-shredded Cabbage ◆ 1 package Sweetner ◆ Salt to taste ◆ 1/4 teaspoon Vinegar (or to taste) ◆ Frozen Dill

Onions with Balsamic Vinegar

Place onions in a bowl. Sprinkle with salt; add vinegar and mint. Toss onions. Allow to stand at least 1 hour before serving.

Ingredients

8 oz. Onions sliced into half-moon shapes ◆ Salt, 3 tablespoons Balsamic Vinegar ◆ 1 tablespoon dried crushed Mint

Oyster Salad

Toss oysters, egg, greens, and celery together. Add allowable portion of mayonnaise.

Ingredients

2 ounces well-drained oysters ◆ 1 hard boiled egg ◆ 1 cup greens ◆ 1 cup finely chopped celery ◆ mayonnaise

Pico de Gallo, Oriental

Shred carrot and zucchini. Chop tomato. Over vegetables, pour rice vinegar, salt, and allowable portion of sesame oil. Refrigerate overnight. Salad will keep up to five days in the refrigerator. Add 3 packets of sweetener for a change. Makes 1 finger salad.

Ingredients

1 carrot, shredded ◆ 1 zucchini, shredded ◆ 1 tomato, chopped ◆ 1/4 cup vinegar ◆ 1/2 to 1 teaspoon of salt, to taste ◆ sesame oil

Pumpkin-Yogurt Unbaked Soufflé

Blend all ingredients. Eat with a spoon. You may put the remaining pumpkin from the 2 c or 4 c can in small containers to freeze or store in the refrigerator for future use.

Ingredients

1/2 c uncooked canned "100% pure pumpkin" ◆ 1 c plain yogurt ◆ nutmeg & cinnamon to taste

Relish

Dice pickles and put in blender. Add other ingredients. Put in jar with cinnamon stick and clove and shut tight. Let marinate at least 24 hours.

Ingredients

1 cup dill pickle ◆ 1 cup vinegar ◆ onion flakes ◆ 1/2 cup diced carrots ◆ 3 packets sweetener substitute

Salad, Chef's Style

Measure out salad vegetables. Add weighed cold cuts, such as ham, turkey, chicken, salami, or soy cold cuts. Top with weighed shredded cheese, such as cheddar, american, or mozarella. Add allowable portion of salad dressing. Sprinkle on favorite abstinent salad spices. Make sure that cold cuts and dressing have sugar as fifth, or lower, ingredient.

Ingredients

2 cups salad ◆ 2 ounces cold cuts ◆ 1 ounce shredded cheese ◆ salad dressing

Salad, Taco Style

Measure out taco-style salad vegetables, such as lettuce, tomato, carrots, etc. Stir cooked ground beef or soy in with cooked onions and tomato sauce. Top salad with cooked meat and onions. Add allowable portion of ranch dressing on top.

Ingredients

2 cups salad ◆ 4 ounces cooked ground beef or 4 ounces cooked ground soy, such as Gimme Lean ◆ 1/2 cup sauteed onions ◆ 2 ounces tomato sauce, taco spices or abstinent seasoned salt ◆ ranch dressing

Salmon Salad

Combine flaked salmon with vegetables. Toss well with allowable portion of mayonnaise. Variation: Use spinach as the greens.

Ingredients

1/2 cup flaked, cold, poached salmon ◆ 1/2 cup greens ◆ 1/2 cup sliced, peeled, and seeded cucumber ◆ 1/2 cup finely cut celery ◆ 1/2 cup finely cut green onions mayonnaise

Sausage Cucumber Salad

Cook sausage in microwave long enough to warm it. Weigh 2 ounces sausage cooked. Measure lunch or dinner portion of cucumbers as salad. Mix sausage and cucumbers with measured portion of cottage cheese. Serve.

Ingredients

1/4 cup cottage cheese ◆ 2 ounces sausage, or soy sausage ◆ several large cucumbers, peeled, sliced, and quartered

Shrimp and Cabbage Salad

Combine celery, cabbage, and tomatoes. Stir in mustard and allowable portion of mayonnaise. Chill for 2 to 3 hours. Add shrimp, salt, and pepper, and serve.

Ingredients

4 oz. cooked, chilled shrimp ◆ 1 cup chopped shredded cabbage ◆ 1/2 cup chopped celery ◆ 1/2 cup sliced tomatoes ◆ 1 tablespoon mustard ◆ mayonnaise ◆ salt and pepper

Shrimp-Cucumber Cups

Wash the cucumbers but do not peel. Cut cucumbers in 3/4-inch slices. Form into little cups by scooping out the cucumber seeds with a melon cutter or small fork. Combine chopped shrimp, salt, mace, and Tabasco. Spray shrimp lightly with zero-calorie butter spray. Stuff cucumbers with shrimp mixture. Place on a platter. Cover with foil or plastic wrap. Chill thoroughly.

Ingredients

3 raw cucumbers ◆ 4 ounces cooked shrimp, chopped finely zero-calorie butter spray ◆ 1/2 teaspoon salt ◆ 1/4 teaspoon mace dash of Tabasco

Simple Raws

Chop and mix.

Ingredients

1 tomato ◆ 2 red peppers, fresh basil (5 leaves) ◆ 1 Equal, black pepper, dried oregano, garlic powder, onion powder ◆ 1 tablespoon olive oil

Soy Bean Dip

Mix everything in a food processor or blender until smooth. When weighing the tomatoes and mushrooms, you may wish to include some of the juices from the tomatoes in your measurement to help the consistency of the dip. Pour the processed or blended mixture into a microwaveable container and heat on high for about 3 minutes (more if your microwave is lower wattage). You can use that time to clean and ready your raw veggies. *Can be fresh (raw) but you should increase your cooking time accordingly.

Ingredients

3 ounces canned soy beans* ◆ 1 ounce grated or shredded soy cheese ◆ 8 ounces canned chopped tomatoes with green chiles (sometimes sold by the brand name RoTel) and drained ◆ canned mushrooms* ◆ 1/4 to 1/2 teaspoon hot red pepper flakes ◆ 1/2 teaspoon garlic powder ◆ 1 teaspoon onion powder ◆ 1/2 teaspoon ground celery seed (celery powder) ◆ 1/2 teaspoon salt (or to taste), ◆ Raw veggies from Lunch Finger Salad or Dinner Salad

Texturized Soy Protein Thai Salad

Combine texturized soy protein with 1/2 cup hot water and unsweetened ketchup. Let stand 5 minutes. Meanwhile, combine soy sauce, vinegar, garlic, red pepper, sweetener, and lemon juice, and set aside. Slice carrots and green onion. Shred cabbage. Combine soy protein mixture with soy sauce mixture in a microwaveable dish. Cover with plastic wrap and microwave on medium-high for 8 minutes, until chunks are tender and liquid is absorbed. Heat a large non-stick skillet or wok sprayed with zero-calorie butter spray. Stir-fry the soy protein for about 3-5 minutes until browned. Add salad veggies to wok and spray them with Pam. Mix with soy protein for about 1 minute or less until they are lightly warmed but still raw. Remove and top with sesame oil, for dressing.

Ingredients

4 ounces chunk style texturized soy protein (these are larger chunks of soy granules, about 1/4 cubed, if you can find them) ◆ 2 cups salad - thinly sliced carrots and regular, or Chinese, cabbage, and green onions, if desired ◆ 1 ounce unsweetened ketchup or tomato sauce with spices ◆ 1 ounce soy sauce ◆ 3 tablespoons vinegar ◆ 1 teaspoon garlic ◆ minced ◆ sweetener ◆ 1/8 - 1/2 teaspoon red pepper ◆ 1 tablespoon lemon juice ◆ 1 tablespoons sesame oil (fat), zero-calorie butter spray

Tomato Broccoli

Clean and cut up the broccoli. Quarter the cherry tomatoes and put on top. Add parsley and salt. Measure salad for lunch or dinner.

Ingredients

1 bunch broccoli ◆ 1 dozen cherry tomatoes ◆ 3 tablespoons minced parsley ◆ salt

Tomato Salad

Arrange tomato slices on a platter; sprinkle with lemon juice. Warm oil in a small pan over medium heat. Add cumin, fennel and chili pepper; cook for 30 seconds. Remove from heat, discard pod and cool. Spoon seasoned oil over tomatoes, sprinkle with cilantro, salt and pepper.

Ingredients

12 to 16 oz. tomatoes, sliced ◆ 1 tablespoon lemon juice ◆ 2 tablespoons olive oil ◆ 1/4 teaspoon ground cumin ◆ 1/4 teaspoon fennel seed ◆ 1 dried red chile pepper ◆ 2 tablespoons chopped fresh cilantro ◆ salt and pepper to taste

Tomatoes and Onion Salad

Slice tomatoes and onion. Toss slices together. Add allowable portion of olive oil, lemon juice, and vinegar. Usually eaten raw with salt and freshly ground pepper, or over broiled meats with allowable portion of mayonnaise.

Ingredients

Fresh, ripe, beefsteak ◆ tomatoes ◆ Young, sweet, Italian onion

Tongue and Spinach Salad

Slice tomatoes and onion. Toss slices together. Add allowable portion of olive oil, lemon juice, and vinegar. Usually eaten raw with salt and freshly ground pepper, or over broiled meats with allowable portion of mayonnaise.

Ingredients

3 1/2 ounces julienne of tongue ◆ 1/2 ounce bacon bits ◆ 2 cups spinach leaves ◆ 1 tablespoon horseradish vinaigrette dressing

Vietnamese Cucumber Salad

Mix all ingredients in a bowl. Weigh, measure and enjoy.

Ingredients

2 Cucumbers ◆ Soy sauce ◆ Fresh mint ◆ Lime juice ◆ Chili garlic sauce (from Asian food market, jar has a green lid and a rooster on the front (ingredients: Chili, Vinegar, Garlic, Salt, Potassium Sorbate and Sodium Bisulfite)

Zucchini Salad

Dice up all 3 raw vegetables, toss with oil, vinegar and sweetener.

Ingredients

21 zucchini squash ◆ 1 carrot ◆ 1 tomato ◆ 1 teaspoon oil ◆ 1 teaspoon rice vinegar ◆ sweetener to taste

Raw Vegetable with Dairy, Soy Protein

3 Raws Salad

MIX and enjoy!

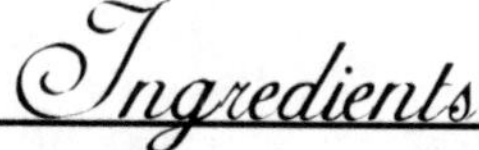

4 oz Yogurt ◆ 2 oz Soy Nuts (mix in at end right before eating) ◆ 3 Raw Vegetables ◆ 1oz Wheat Germ (toasted is best) ◆ Brown mustard

Cauliflower Bacon Slaw

Puree cottage cheese into a smooth paste. In a large bowl add cottage cheese, mayonnaise, onion powder, salt, pepper and sweetener and mix. Add remaining ingredients and mix until vegetables are well coated.

Ingredients

3 oz. chopped romaine, spinach or red leaf lettuce ◆ 9 oz. chopped cauliflower ◆ 1/4-3/8 cup cottage cheese ◆ 1/2 to 1 oz. turkey or pork bacon crumbled ◆ 1 tablespoon mayonnaise ◆ 1/2 to 1 teaspoon onion powder ◆ 1/2 to 1 teaspoon salt ◆ 1/4 teaspoon pepper, sweetener to taste

Chili

Puree cottage cheese into a smooth paste. In a large bowl add cottage cheese, mayonnaise, onion powder, salt, pepper and sweetener and mix. Add remaining ingredients and mix until vegetables are well coated.

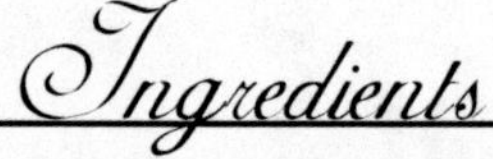

2 oz TVP (weighed first, then you add water to reconstitute) ◆ 1 oz Black Soybeans ◆ 2 oz Tomato Sauce ◆ UnKetchup (free condiment- check w/ your sponsor) ◆ Chili Powder ◆ Cumin ◆ 2 Equal ◆ 1 oz Soy Cheese (to melt on top)

Cucumbers and Cream

Whip cottage cheese, herbs, and salt to taste, in blender. Spread on cucumbers and refrigerate. Serve cold.

Ingredients

1/2 cup cottage cheese ◆ 3 raw, sliced cucumbers ◆ 2 teaspoons of fresh herbs (dill or chives) ◆ salt

Salmon Salad

Combine flaked salmon with vegetables. Toss well with allowable portion of mayonnaise. Variation: Use spinach as the greens.

Ingredients

1/2 cup flaked cold poached salmon ◆ 1/2 cup greens ◆ 1/2 cup sliced, peeled, and seeded cucumber ◆ 1/2 cup finely cut celery ◆ 1/2 cup finely cut green onions ◆ mayonnaise

Sausage Cucumber Salad

Cook sausage in microwave long enough to warm it. Weigh 2 ounces sausage cooked. Measure lunch or dinner portion of cucumbers as salad. Mix sausage and cucumbers with measured portion of cottage cheese. Serve.

Ingredients

1/4 cup cottage cheese ◆ 2 ounces sausage, or soy sausage ◆ several large cucumbers, peeled, sliced, and quartered

Tried and True Tuna Salad

Mix and enjoy.

Ingredients

4 oz Tuna ◆ 1 cup mixed chopped Celery/Onion/Parsley/Dill (no sugar) ◆ Pickle (if you like) ◆ 1 tablespoon Mayonnaise

Vegetable Salad

Bake pepperoni in microwave for 2-3 minutes. It gets light and crispy. Weigh after baking. Sprinkle with onion and/or garlic powder

Ingredients

16 oz. Raw Salad Veggies ◆ 3 oz. Roasted (salted, if desired) Soy Nuts ◆ 1 oz. sliced Pepperoni ◆ 1 oz. Wheat Germ

Vegetable Salad

Bake pepperoni in microwave for 2-3 minutes. It gets light and crispy. Weigh after baking. Sprinkle with onion and/or garlic powder

Ingredients

16 oz. Raw Salad Veggies ◆ 3 oz. Roasted (salted, if desired) Soy Nuts ◆ 1 oz. sliced Pepperoni ◆ 1 oz. Wheat Germ

Protein

Abstinent BBQ Turkey Burgers

Add all ingredients in a bowl. Mix well. Use generous helpings of spices and bbq sauce. Form into burgers. Cook as you would hamburger either on a grill or in a frying pan (I usually either spray pan with butter flavored sprayor add water to bottom of pan so burgers don't stick. Cook until done.

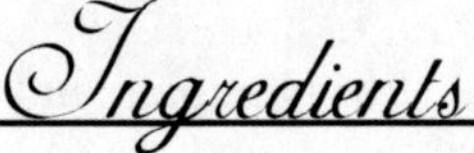

1 package ground turkey ◆ onion powder ◆ garlic powder ◆ salt ◆ pepper ◆ Texas Best "originial recipe" BBQ sauce (***Caution: All other varieties of Texas Best are not abstinent.)

Abstinent Turkey Burgers

Add all ingredients in a bowl. Mix well. Use generous helpings of spices and barbecue sauce. Either on a grill or in a frying pan form into burgers and cook as you would hamburger. Cook until done.

Ingredients

1 package ground turkey ◆ onion powder ◆ garlic powder ◆ salt ◆ pepper ◆ Texas Best "original recipe" BBQ sauce
Caution: All other varieties of Texas Best are not abstinent.

Amish Chicken

Preheat oven to 350° F. Stir together soy flour, garlic powder, white pepper, salt, paprika, and parsley in a large bowl. Rinse chicken and lightly pat dry. Dredge chicken in soy flour mixture, shaking off excess, and set aside. In a large ceramic casserole or heavy roasting pan, mix the soymilk and soy cream cheese over a low flame until they have completely blended. Lay the chicken pieces in the pan in a single layer. Bake in the middle of the oven 1½ hours or until skin is golden and crisp.

Ingredients

½ cup soy flour ◆ 2 tsp garlic powder ◆ 1 tsp white pepper ◆ 1 Tb salt ◆ 2 tsp paprika ◆ 2 Tb finely chopped fresh parsley ◆ 1 chicken, quartered, or 2 lbs boneless chicken pieces, skin on ◆ ½-1 cup soy milk ◆ ¼ cup soy cream cheese

Bacon-Wrapped Hors d-Oeuvre

If using little sausages, blanch for 4 minutes in boiling water. If using crabmeat, select chunks of backfin from blue crabs or legs of Dungeness. If using shrimp, marinate them in soy sauce for one hour first. If using chicken livers, cut them into sections large enough to be rolled in bacon. Wrap meat in partially cooked bacon strips and secure with toothpicks. Place on rack in broiling pan or shallow roasting pan and broil 5 inches from broiling unit, or bake in oven at 450F. Turn once if necessary. Remove toothpicks before weighing. Weigh 4 ounces and serve.

Ingredients

little sausages ◆ crabmeat ◆ shrimp, or chicken livers ◆ Bacon (no sugar in ingredients)

Balsamic vinegar Chicken

Heat the oil in a large flameproof casserole or baking dish over a medium-low flame. Sprinkle the chicken breasts with salt and pepper. When the oil is hot, add the garlic (cut side down) and fry gently. Add the vinegar, thyme, black peppercorns, and bay leaves (and a few Tb water if necessary). Lay the chicken breasts evenly across the casserole. Reduce heat to very, very low (using a heat-diffuser pad for electric ranges, if you have one) and simmer, uncovered, for about 1 hour, or until the liquid has evaporated. Remove from heat and leave to cool to room temperature before serving. (This is designed to be served cold.)

Ingredients

1 lb boneless chicken breasts ◆ 1 Tb olive oil ◆ 1 tsp truffle oil ◆ 1 Tb balsamic vinegar ◆ 2 Tb good white vinegar ◆ 1 whole head garlic unpeeled and cut in half horizontally ◆ 1 Tb onion powder ◆ 2 sprigs fresh thyme ◆ 3 bay leaves ◆ 7 black peppercorns ◆ salt and freshly ground black pepper

Beef Slices with Rosemary

Heat a large heavy frying pan and add the oil and garlic. Pan-fry the meat on both sides quickly over medium-high heat. Salt and pepper the meat and remove it to a heated serving platter. Add the rosemary to the pan along with 1/4 cup water. Deglaze the pan and pour the resulting sauce over the meat.

Ingredients

1 Tb olive oil ◆ 2 cloves garlic, coarsely chopped ◆ 1 lb lean roast beef sliced quite thin ◆ salt and freshly ground black pepper to taste ◆ 1 Tb chopped fresh rosemary

Beef Tenderloin

Combine everything but the meat in a small bowl. Line a baking pan with foil and place the roast on it. Spread the sauce over the roast, covering it as thoroughly as possible. Broil at 500° F for 30-35 minutes.

Ingredients

1 beef tenderloin, beef roast, London broil, etc ◆ 2-4 cloves garlic, pressed ◆ salt ◆ 2 tablespoons mustard ◆ 1 tablespoon parsley ◆ 2 tablespoons basil ◆ 2 tablespoons marjoram ◆ 2 tablespoons thyme ◆ ground pepper ◆ 1 tablespoons olive oil ◆ 1 tablespoon liquid sweetener

Beef, Savory Meatballs

Heat oven to 350°F. In a mixing bowl, combine sirloin, wheat germ, parsley and seasoning. If necessary, add a little water to beef mixture to hold it together. Roll into meat balls. Place on an broiling rack, sprayed with zero-calorie butter spray, and bake 15 minutes.

Ingredients

4 ounces ground sirloin ◆ 1/8 cup wheat germ ◆ abstinent Italian or pizza seasoning ◆ zero-calorie butter spray

Cajun Prime Rib

Place the roast, standing on the rib bones, in a very large roasting pan. Then make several dozen punctures through the silver skin so seasoning can permeate the meat. Pour a very generous, even layer of black pepper over the top of the meat until evenly covered; repeat procedure with garlic powder, then salt. Refrigerate 24 hours. Bake ribs in a 550° oven until fat is brown and crispy, about 35 minutes. Remove from oven and cool slightly. Refrigerate until very well chilled, about 3 hours. Scrape off seasonings, then slice between ribs into 6 steaks; trim the cooked surface from the two pieces that were on the end. Coat with seasoning mix and blacken in a cast-iron skillet, or grill.

Ingredients

Seasoning Mix: 1 Tb + 2 tsp salt ◆ 1 Tb + 2 tsp white pepper ◆ 1 Tb + 2 tsp whole fennel seeds ◆ 1 Tb + 3/4 tsp black pepper ◆ 2 1/2 tsp dry mustard ◆ 2 1/2 tsp cayenne, Roast: 1 (4-bone) prime rib of beef roast about 10 1/2 lbs ◆ 1/4 cup black pepper ◆ 1/4 cup garlic powder ◆ 1/4 cup salt

Chicken Alfredo

Place chicken in a single layer in a glass baking dish and bake at 350° F for 30-40 minutes or until well-done but not dried out. Place chicken in a single layer in a glass baking dish and bake at 350° F for 30-40 minutes or until well-done but not dried out. Remove chicken from pan, allow to cool, and cut into bite-sized pieces. Drain off excess chicken fat but leave some in the pan. Place pan over a burner on the stove and sauté the chopped garlic. Add 1 cup water, bring to a boil, reduce heat, and simmer for 10 minutes, scraping up scrunchens from the bottom of the pan. Add soy cream cheese and soy parmesan and cook, stirring, until well-blended. Add salt and pepper to taste and return chicken to pan. Allow to heat through.

Ingredients

1 lb boneless chicken ◆ 2 cloves garlic ◆ 1/2 cup soy parmesan ◆ 1/4 cup soy cream cheese ◆ salt and pepper

Chicken 'Almondine'

Combine soy flour, salt, pepper and onion powder. Dust the mixture onto the chicken breasts. Heat 2 Tb of the oil in a heavy skillet. Slowly brown the chicken breasts on both sides. Add the lemon juice and 1/2 cup water, deglaze the pan, and season with salt and pepper to taste. Cover the pan and simmer gently until the chicken is tender (10-15 minutes). Remove the chicken from the skillet. Add the remaining oil and the garlic and stir to mix thoroughly with the existing sauce. Add vinegar, stir, and return the chicken to the skillet. Sprinkle with chopped parsley.

Ingredients

6 boneless, skinless chicken breasts ◆ 1 Tb white vinegar ◆ 2 Tb lemon juice ◆ 1 Tb almond oil (or walnut oil or hazelnut oil if you prefer) ◆ 2 tsp finely chopped fresh parsley ◆ 2 Tb soy flour ◆ salt and pepper ◆ 1 tsp garlic pressed ◆ 1 Tb onion powder

Chicken Bog

Boil chicken with salt in 6 cups water until tender. (About 1 hour.) Remove chicken, let cool and remove bones. Chop meat in bite-sized pieces. Skim off fat from juices. Measure 3 1/2 cups of this broth into a 6-qt saucepan. Add soy nuggets, chicken pieces and smoked sausage, herb seasoning and poultry seasoning. Cook these ingredients for 30 minutes. Let come to a boil and turn to low, keeping covered the entire time. If mixture is too juicy, cook uncovered until desired consistency. If you use already-cut or boneless chicken, reduce the boiling time accordingly.

Ingredients

1 3-lb chicken ◆ 1 Tb salt ◆ 1 cup soy nuggets ◆ 1/2 lb smoked sausage sliced ◆ 1 Tb onion powder ◆ 2 Tb mixed herbs ◆ 1 Tb poultry seasoning if you can find an abstinent variety

Chicken Breasts Diane

Wash chicken breasts, pat dry, and sprinkle with salt and pepper. Heat olive oil in a skillet and fry chicken breasts over high heat for 4 minutes on each side. Transfer chicken to a warm serving platter, lower heat, and add the chives, lemon juice, parsley and mustard to the pan. Cook, whisking constantly, for 15 seconds. Add 2 Tb water and stir until the sauce is smooth. Return chicken to the pan and cook until just heated through.

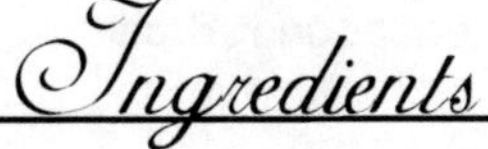

2 large boneless chicken breast halves ◆ 1 Tb olive oil ◆ 1/2 tsp salt ◆ 1/2 tsp black pepper ◆ 3 Tb chopped fresh parsley ◆ 3 Tb chopped fresh chives ◆ 2 Tb mustard ◆ 1 Tb lemon juice

Chicken Breasts, Sauteed

Spray skillet with zero-calorie butter spray. Add soy sauce and garlic powder to skillet. Add chicken breasts. Cook until no longer pink. Measure 4 ounces and serve.

Ingredients

4 boneless skinless chicken breasts ◆ zero-calorie spray butter ◆ 1 teaspoon soy sauce ◆ 1/4 teaspoon garlic powder

Chicken Chaat

Wash and cut the chicken into one inch pieces. Spray pan with zero-calorie butter spray and heat. Add garlic and salt. Stri-fry the garlic and salt until it is light brown. Add chicken pieces. Stir-fry for 5-6 minutes, stirring constantly. Add the masala powders. Stir for another 3-4 minutes. Check to see if the chicken is tender. Remove from heat. Weigh 4 ounces and serve. Option: Top chicken with 1 tsp. lemon juice.

Ingredients

1 boneless chicken breast ◆ 2-3 cloves garlic, peeled and chopped ◆ zero-calorie butter spray ◆ 1 1/2 teaspoons dry coriander powder ◆ 1/4 teaspoon turmeric powder ◆ 1/4- 1/2 teaspoon red chili powder ◆ salt

Chicken Cutlets (Schnitzel)

Butterfly chicken breast. Season to taste. Dunk chicken in the egg (wet hand) and then coat in TVP (dry hand :).Fry at low to medium heat until cooked. Best eaten when done, does not re-heat as well.

Ingredients

Boneless chicken breast ◆ Frying oil ◆ 1 egg scrambled in a dish (large enough to contain the chicken pieces) ◆ TVP in a plate (large enough to place the chicken in) ◆ Seasonings to taste

Chicken Parmesan

Heat oven to 400° F. Line a 15 x 10 x 1-inch baking pan with foil. Brush chicken breasts with olive oil. Combine remaining ingredients in a bowl. Roll the chicken breasts in the soy Parmesan mixture and place into pan. Pour remaining soy over chicken. Bake 20-25 minutes.

Ingredients

6 boneless skinless chicken breast halves (about 2 lb.) ◆ 1 Tb olive oil ◆ 1/2 cup soy parmesan ◆ 1/4 cup soy granules ◆ 1 tsp dried oregano leaves ◆ 1 tsp parsley flakes ◆ 1/4 tsp paprika ◆ 1/4 tsp salt ◆ 1/4 tsp black pepper

Chicken Piccata

Combine soy flour, salt and pepper in a shallow dish. Dredge chicken breasts in flour mixture; shake off excess. Heat vegetable oil in a large, heavy sauté pan over medium heat. Add chicken breasts. Cook about 3 minutes per side, until tender and opaque. Remove and keep warm. Add vinegar to pan juices. Cook 1 minute, scraping up brown bits from bottom of pan. Add lemon juice and heat to boiling. Return chicken to pan and cook until sauce thickens slightly, about 3 minutes. Add chopped fresh parsley just before serving.

Ingredients

1/2 cup soy flour ◆ 1 tsp salt ◆ 1/2 tsp freshly ground pepper ◆ 2 lbs skinless boneless chicken breast halves pounded to 1/4-inch thickness ◆ 3 Tb vegetable oil ◆ 2 Tb white vinegar ◆ 1 Tb lemon juice, chopped fresh parsley

Chicken Piccata

Melt allowable portion of margarine in a small skillet. Add onion, diced chicken, and soy sauce; toss until warm. Mix allowable portion of salad dressing and ketchup together. Add bacon, salsa/dressing mixture, and finally chicken and onion to salad.

Ingredients

4 ounces combination diced, cooked chicken breast and cooked bacon ◆ 1/2 cup onion (cooked in microwave 8 minutes) ◆ 2 cups salad, ranch dressing ◆ 1 tablespoon soy sauce ◆ 2 tablespoons diet ketchup with onion and chili powder to taste ◆ margarine

Chicken Salad

Melt allowable portion of margarine in a small skillet. Add onion, diced chicken, and soy sauce; toss until warm. Mix allowable portion of salad dressing and ketchup together. Add bacon, salsa/dressing mixture, and finally chicken and onion to salad.

Ingredients

4 ounces combination diced, cooked chicken breast and cooked bacon ◆ 1/2 cup onion (cooked in microwave 8 minutes) ◆ 2 cups salad ◆ ranch dressing ◆ 1 tablespoon soy sauce ◆ 2 tablespoons diet ketchup with onion and chili powder to taste ◆ margarine

Chicken with 50 cloves of garlic

Place olive oil in a heavy pot which can be tightly covered. Add 1/3 of garlic and 1/3 of all remaining ingredients, including chicken. Add a second third of garlic and of the other ingredients. Add remaining chicken and remaining ingredients. Then cover pot tightly and place in a 375° F oven for about 1 hour and 15 minutes. The chicken will not brown, but will be moist and succulent. Purée the softened garlic cloves and sauce before serving.

Ingredients

1 Tb olive oil ◆ 40-60 (that's right!) plump garlic cloves peeled ◆ 2 lbs boneless, skinless chicken thighs ◆ 1/2 cup chopped parsley ◆ 1 tsp dried tarragon ◆ 1 Tb salt ◆ 1 tsp white pepper ◆ 1/2 tsp ground allspice ◆ 1/4 tsp cinnamon ◆ 3 Tb white vinegar

Chicken, Roasted with Rub

Mix all spices together in small bowl. Using a whole chicken fryer, carefully separate the skin from the meat and sprinkle rub in between the skin and meat. Gently rub the outer skin of the chicken where the spices were placed. Refrigerate the chicken for 1 hour. Roast in oven at 350 degrees until internal temp is 160 degrees. If available, rotisserie chicken for 1 1/4 hours. Measure 4 ounces and serve.

Ingredients

1 whole chicken fryer ◆ 2 teaspoons coriander, ground ◆ 2 teaspoons cumin, ground ◆ 2 teaspoons garlic powder ◆ 2 teaspoons marjoram, ground ◆ 2 teaspoons nutmeg, ground ◆ 2 teaspoons onion powder ◆ 1 teaspoon salt ◆ 2 teaspoons thyme, ground

Chili

Sauté ground beef, drain black soybeans mix together. Add all spices, along with 2 oz tomato sauce. Simmer on low heat for about 15 minutes.

Ingredients

4 oz Black Soybeans and Ground Beef ◆ 2 oz Tomato Sauce ◆ 1 tablespoon Chili Powder ◆ Onion Flakes ◆ 2 Equal ◆ 1 tablespoon Red Pepper

Chicken, Sunset Barbecue

If you are using an oven broiler, heat oven (not broiler) to 450°F/200°C. Rinse chicken and pat dry. Set chicken on grill for 20 minutes, not directly over heat. Cover the grill, and open the vents or place chicken in a foil-lined pan, and roast for 20 minutes. While the chicken is pre-cooking, whisk the remaining ingredients together in a small bowl. If you are using an oven broiler, remove chicken from oven, and pre-heat the broiler. Brush half of this mixture on top of the chicken. Return chicken to heat for 5 minutes. Turn chicken and baste underside with the remaining sauce. Cook until meat is no longer pink at the bone in the thickest part (about 5 minutes). The mustard coating should not be burnt.

Ingredients

2-3 pounds chicken pieces, skin removed ◆ 1 teaspoon liquid sweetener ◆ 2 tablespoons dijon-style mustard ◆ 1 tablespoon worcestershire sauce ◆ 1 teaspoon grated fresh ginger ◆ 1 clove garlic, pressed ◆ salt and pepper

Chimichurri Chicken

Put all ingredients for chimichurri sauce into blender or food processor and blend until smooth. Put the sauce into a glass bowl or plastic food bag. Add chicken; turn to coat well. Marinate in the refrigerator at least 1 hour and up to 4 hours. Prepare charcoal grill or heat broiler. While grill heats, soak wooden skewers in water at least 20 minutes so they don't burn. Thread chicken onto skewers. Grill, basting occasionally with the sauce, until chicken is no longer pink and edges are slightly golden, 10 to 15 minutes. Serve immediately.

Ingredients

Chimichurri sauce: 1 Tb olive oil ◆ 1/2 cup fresh curly parsley chopped ◆ 1 tablespoon fresh lemon juice ◆ 1 teaspoon cracked black pepper ◆ 6 cloves garlic ◆ 1/2 teaspoon salt. Poultry: 1 lb boneless skinless chicken breast cut into 1-inch wide strips

Chipotle-Mustard Chicken

Whisk all ingredients except chicken together in an airtight container with a little water. Marinate the chicken for at least one hour. Grill over hot coals or bake in a 400° F oven until tender and just starting to brown.This has a lot of zip, but is not overwhelmingly hot.

Ingredients

2 cloves garlic pressed ◆ 1 tsp salt ◆ 1 tsp (or more) liquid sweetener ◆ 1 Tb apple cider vinegar ◆ 1 Tb Dijon mustard ◆ 1 Tb chipotle purée ◆ 1 Tb ground mustard ◆ 2 tsp dried thyme ◆ 2 tsp dried tarragon ◆ 1 lb boneless skinless chicken breasts or thighs

Chocolate Layer Cake with Soy Nut Butter Filling

Put 2 oz. soy flour into a microwaveable bowl, add a bit of powdered cinnamon and ginger. Add 1 1/2 packets of sweet 'n low (equal doesn't work because when cooked it loses its sweetnesss). Add about a third to a half can of diet chocolate soda (you can use cream if you can't find chocolate soda). Add chocolate extract and coconut extracts to the mixture (you can add others to your liking -- almond, vanilla, orange, lemon, butterscotch, etc.) Stir with a fork unto all the flour is absorbed by the liquid. As it is absorbed, decide if you need more liquid to reach a thick pancake batter consistency. Microwave for 8 minutes (times vary depending on your microwave). Put in frig or freezer to cool. The cooler the better. Slice the cake into layers - two, three or four layers. Spread 2 oz. soy nut butter to the layers.Variation: Instead of soy nut butter, you can add soy cream cheese, sprinkled with ginger and equal, or with other condiments and/or extracts.

Ingredients

2 oz. Soy flower, powered cinnamon and ginger, sweet and low ◆ 1 can diet chocolate soda; chocolate extract, coconut extract (and/or any others to your liking) ◆ 1 oz. Soynut butter

Clams, Steamed

Wash clams thoroughly, scrubbing under cold, running water. Place in large kettle or Dutch oven, on rack, so clams don't touch the bottom. Sprinkle with seasonings. Add water, cover tightly, and bring to boiling point. Steam just until the shells open, about 5 minutes. Discard any that do not open. Remove from shells. Weigh 4 ounces. Serve with allowable portion of butter.

Ingredients

3 pounds clams in shell ◆ 1 1/2 cups water, abstinent seafood seasoning 1/4 tsp. thyme, optional ◆ 1-2 sprigs parsley, salt and pepper, butter

Crab Louis

Mix crab, tomato sauce, and allowable portion of mayonnaise together. Serve on top of 2 cups lettuce. This is best made with Dungeness crab, but lump crabmeat is almost as good. Meat from lobster tails may also be used. Variation: 1/4 cup crab and 1 hard-boiled egg, sliced.

Ingredients

1/2 cup crab ◆ 2 cups shredded lettuce
◆ 2 ounces tomato sauce or chili sauce, mayonnaise

Coriander Lamb

Dice the meat into bite-sized cubes and soak in warm water for 2-3 minutes. Mix the paprika, ground coriander, salt, crushed garlic, onion powder, and cayenne pepper with the vinegar. Drain the lamb and add to the marinade. Marinate in the refrigerator for 6- 24 hours. Heat the oil in a large heavy saucepan. Add the black mustard seeds and stir a few times. Then add the ginger, cumin seeds, red chillies and turmeric powder. Increase the heat and fry this masala for a couple of minutes. Add the marinated lamb to the masala and mix well. At this point you have two options, either to cook the meat on the stove or to bake it. Stovetop cooking takes less time but requires fairly constant stirring. Leave meat in saucepan, reduce heat, cover, and stew over a low to medium flame for about 45 minutes. Add water if the sauce gets too dry and begins to stick. For baking, transfer meat and sauce to an ovenproof casserole, cover it, and bake for 1 1/2 hours at 95° C . Check occasionally, though you are unlikely to need to add any water to the sauce. Finally, prepare and wash the fresh coriander in cold water. Only the leaves and the tender stems should be retained. Chop coarsely and mix well just before serving. If you don't have any fresh coriander, use dried cilantro. Note: this works with beef, as well. The tougher the meat you start out with, the longer you should marinate it and the longer you should stew it.

Ingredients

1 1/2 lbs stewing lamb trimmed of fat and cut into bite-sized pieces ◆ 6 cloves garlic pressed ◆ 1 Tb ground coriander ◆ 1/2 tsp cayenne pepper ◆ 1 Tb onion powder ◆ 2 Tb malt vinegar ◆ 1 Tb paprika ◆ 1 Tb salt ◆ 2 Tb mustard oil ◆ 1 1/2 tsp cumin seeds ◆ 1/4 tsp turmeric ◆ 1/2 tsp black mustard seeds ◆ 1 tsp grated ginger ◆ 2 dried red peppers soaked and chopped ◆ 4 oz fresh coriander (cilantro)

Crab Salad

Mix greens, celery, and onion. Stir in mustard and allowable portion of mayonnaise. Chill for 2 to 3 hours. Top with crabmeat and serve.

Ingredients

1/2 cup crabmeat ◆ 1 1/4 cup lettuce greens ◆ 1/2 cup finely cut celery ◆ 1/4 cup finely cut onion, mustard, mayonnaise

Crockpot BBQ Ribs

Cut a rack of ribs so they fit in the crock pot. Add about 3/4 bottle of Texas Best Original Recipe. Set on low...let slow cook overnight.(or about 8 hrs). The meat will fall off the bone and you can weigh it after cooked.

Ingredients

Rack of ribs ◆ Texas Best "original recipe" BBQ sauce

Curried Chicken Liver Paté

Heat the oil in a deep, heavy frying pan over medium heat. Sauté the chicken livers with the spices until they are barely pink inside, about 10 minutes. Remove from heat and purée in a large food processor until smooth. Pour paté into a container that will hold it comfortably and refrigerate until firm, at least 3 hours. Best the day after it is made, but actually just fine straight from the food processor.

Ingredients

1 lb chicken livers rinsed and trimmed ◆ 1 Tb onion powder ◆ 2 tsp curry powder ◆ 2 tsp paprika, salt to taste ◆ ½ tsp black pepper ◆ 2 Tb extra virgin olive oil

Deep fried Tofu

Put soy flour and garlic salt or Chinese spices in one bowl and 2 beaten eggs in another. Slice tofu into little sticks (like steak fries). Dip them in the egg and then the flour to "bread" them. Fry until golden brown.

Ingredients

soy flour ◆ garlic salt or Chinese spices ◆ 2 beaten eggs, extra firm tofu

Dressing, Yogurt and Onion

Mix together and chill. Makes 1 protein.

Ingredients

1 cup lowfat, plain yogurt ◆ 1/2 ounce onion soup mix (1/2 an envelope)

Dressing, Yogurt Dill

Mix together and chill. Makes 1 protein.

Ingredients

1 cup plain, lowfat yogurt ◆ 1/8 teaspoon onion powder ◆ 1 teaspoon lemon juice ◆ 1/2 teaspoon crushed dill weed ◆ 1/4 teaspoon dry mustard ◆ 1/8 teaspoon garlic powder

Easy Meatball Paprikash

Combine pork, veal, salt, onion powder, and fennel seeds in a large bowl or food processor; blend well. Shape into 1 1/2" balls. Heat oil in 12" skillet over medium-high heat; add meatballs and cook about 12 minutes, turning frequently until well browned on all sides. Using a slotted spoon, remove meatballs to plate. Add paprika, tomato paste, and about 1/2 cup water, and stir to mix well. Increase heat to high; bring to a boil. Return meatballs to pan. Reduce heat and simmer, covered, for 10 minutes, until meatballs are cooked through. Uncover and stir soy milk into meatball mixture. Cook gently until sauce thickens.

Ingredients

1 lb combined ground pork and veal ◆ 1 Tb fennel seeds ◆ 1 tsp salt ◆ 1 Tb vegetable oil ◆ 1 Tb onion powder ◆ 2 Tb paprika ◆ 2 Tb tomato paste ◆ 1 cup soy milk ◆ 2 Tb chopped fresh parsley

Egg Custard

Whisk together first 4 ingredients. Pour into 4 individual oven proof glass or corning ware bowls. Sprinkle with nutmeg. Put bowls in a cake pan and pour boiling water around the bowls to about 1 inch from top of bowls. Bake at 350 degrees for 45 minuts or until firm.

Ingredients

4 eggs beaten ◆ 2 cups of scalded fat-free milk ◆ 4 to 6 packets of Sweet N Low ◆ 1 teaspoon vanilla flavoring, nutmeg

Egg Custard, Coconut-Flavored

Mix in aluminum loaf pan or ramekin. Bake 450 for 15 minutes Reduce oven to 325, and cook for 35 minutes, or until knife comes out clean. Cool in fridge. Add fruit on top if serving at Breakfast.

Ingredients

1 egg ◆ 1 cup milk ◆ sugar-free, alcohol-free coconut extract or coconut coffee syrup ◆ sweetener ◆ pinch of salt (to bring out the sweet flavor)

Egg Omelette with Fish (LOX or Whitefish)

Cut the smoked fish into small pieces. Heat in the sauté-omelet pan to use some of the oils from the fish to naturally season the pan. Crack open the egg and scramble or keep flat and fold over when ready to make a solid omelet.

Ingredients

1 egg ◆ 1 oz smoked fish

Egg Salad

Chop eggs roughly, or push them through the large-holed side of a four sided box grater. In a mixing bowl, mix eggs with allowable portion of mayonnaise, mustard, salt, and pepper into with a wooden spoon. Stir in chopped celery and tomato.

Ingredients

2 hardboiled eggs ◆ 2 cups chopped tomatoes and celery ◆ mayonnaise ◆ 1 tablespoon Dijon mustard ◆ 1/2 teaspoon salt ◆ 1/4 teaspoon pepper

Eggs and Ricotta, Scrambled

Beat the egg together with the ricotta, vanilla , salt, and sweetener, adding a small amount of water if necessary. Spray zero-calorie butter spray, heavily in an omelet pan, over low heat. Pour in egg mixture and cook gently, stirring frequently, until the eggs are just done.

Ingredients

1 egg ◆ 1/4 cup ricotta cheese ◆ 1 teaspoon vanilla ◆ pinch salt ◆ sweetener ◆ zero-calorie butter spray

Eggs, Hard Boiled

Place eggs in pot on stovetop. Cover eggs with 1 inch, or 3 cm, of water. Turn heat on high. Let them come to a real rolling boil. Reduce to a simmer and let them cook for 10 to 12 minutes. Plunge into cold water at once. This prevents green yolks and makes removing the shell easier. If you stir eggs about during cooking, it will help keep the yolks centered. These are great for travel!

Ingredients

2 eggs

Eggs, Scrambled

Crack eggs in small bowl. Add water, salt, and Tabasco. Beat lightly with a fork. Use a 10-inch skillet, preferably Teflon-coated. Spray with zero-calorie spray butter. Place pan over low heat. Add the egg mixture. Let them heat up, and increase heat slightly. Use wooden spoon or plastic spatula to gently scrape bottom of skillet. Scrape eggs into solid masses as they cook. Serve at once.

Ingredients

2 eggs ◆ 2 teaspoons water ◆ 1/4 teaspoon salt ◆ dash of Tabasco ◆ zero-calorie spray butter

Eggs, Soft Boiled

Place eggs in pot on stovetop. Cover eggs with 1 inch, or 3 cm, of water. Turn heat on high. Let them come to a real rolling boil. Reduce to a simmer and let them cook for 3 minutes for soft eggs and 4 minutes for firmer eggs. Plunge into cold water at once. This prevents green yolks and makes removing the shell easier. If you stir eggs about during cooking, it will help keep the yolks centered.

Ingredients

2 eggs

Egyptian Stewed Beef

Heat oil in a large, thick-bottomed saucepan. Add the beef cubes and brown on all sides. Add the onion powder and stir to coat. Stir in the tomato paste, blending it well into the fat. Add a small quantity of water if necessary. Add nutmeg, cinnamon, lemon juice, salt and pepper, and bring to a boil. Cover the pan and simmer gently 1 hour; remove lid and continue simmering to reduce liquid. Meat should be very tender and sauce quite thick.

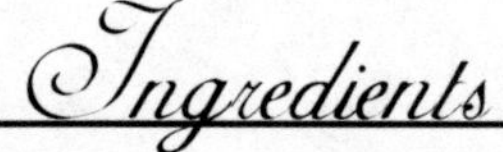

2 lbs beef, cubed ◆ 3 Tb tomato paste ◆ 1 Tb onion powder ◆ 1 Tb oil ◆ 1/4 tsp nutmeg ◆ 1/2 tsp cinnamon ◆ 2 Tb lemon juice ◆ salt and pepper

Fiery Chicken Chili

Heat oil in a large, heavy skillet and add dried hot peppers and garlic. When they begin to change color, add chicken pieces and stir-fry quickly until browned. Add tomato paste, spices, 1 1/2 cups water, and bay leaf. Bring to a boil, reduce heat, and simmer for 10 minutes. Add soybeans (and more water if necessary) and simmer another 20 minutes. How hot this is depends on how much chili powder and/or cayenne you use.

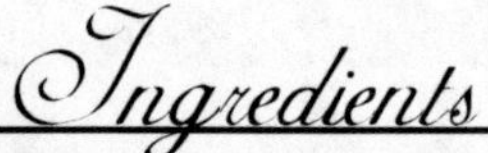

1 lb chicken cut into bite-sized cubes ◆ 1 Tb olive oil ◆ 4 cloves garlic thinly sliced ◆ 2 dried hot red peppers ◆ 1 Tb onion powder ◆ 2 Tb chili powder ◆ 1 tsp cayenne pepper ◆ 1 tsp ground cumin ◆ 2 tsp ground coriander ◆ 1/2 tsp salt ◆ 3 Tb tomato paste ◆ 1 bay leaf ◆ 1 can white soybeans drained (or about 3/4 cup dried soybeans soaked and boiled

Fish in Soy Ginger Sauce

Combine soy sauce and ginger to make ginger sauce. Steam 4 ounces fish and top with sauce.

Ingredients

4 ounces fish ◆ soy sauce ◆ freshly grated ginger

Fish With Spices Recipe

I get spice rubs from Dean and Deluca in Manhattan. I take a salmon filet and this could work with any fish and rub any of the rubs all over it. Cover and refrigerate for 24 hours. Then I spray a pan with non-stick and fry or I wrap in aluminum foil and grill on my gas grill. Fabulous! I also add spices to soy flour then I dredge the fish in the soy flour and bake the same as before sometimes the soy adds a crust to the fish.

Ingredients

Fish ◆ Spice Rubs

Frito de Cordero

Cut the lamb into bite-sized chunks. Trim off the excess fat and any gristle. Heat the oil in a wide saucepan. Add the bay leaf and garlic and fry until the garlic is golden. Discard the bay leaf. Take the pan off the heat and stir the paprika, onion powder, and chili powder into the oil, followed by the meat. Return to a gentle heat and pour in the vinegar. Season and add the thyme. Cover tightly and cook over a very low heat, stirring occasionally, until the meat is tender (10-15 minutes for leg meat, longer for stew meat). Stir in the soy flour and simmer for another 5 minutes, by which time the sauce should be thick and moist, not runny.

Ingredients

2 lbs boned leg of lamb or lamb stew meat ◆ 1 Tb olive oil ◆ 1 Tb onion powder ◆ 4 - 5 cloves garlic sliced ◆ 1 bay leaf ◆ 1 tsp Spanish paprika (pimenton) ◆ pinch of chili powder ◆ 3 Tb balsamic vinegar ◆ salt and pepper ◆ 1 sprig of fresh thyme ◆ 1 Tb soy flour

Greek Roast Chicken

Combine lemon juice, vinegar, olive oil, and spices in a small bowl. Place the chicken in a foil-lined roasting pan. If you are using a whole chicken, rub the mixture all over the chicken, inside and out. If you are using chicken breasts or cut up chicken pieces, pour the marinade over the chicken and mix well. Allow chicken to stand at room temperature for at least 30 minutes. Preheat oven to 350° F/180° C. Bake chicken for 1 ½ to 2 hours if using a whole chicken, and about 45 minutes if you are using chicken pieces. Be careful not to let the chicken dry out.

Ingredients

1 small roasting chicken or 3 lbs chicken pieces skin on ◆ 2 Tb lemon juice ◆ 1 Tb balsamic vinegar ◆ 1Tb Greek olive oil ◆ 1 tsp salt ◆ ½ tsp pepper ◆ 1 tsp oregano

Grey Sheet Meat Loaf/Meatballs

Combine all ingredients in a bowl and mix thoroughly. For meat loaf, place in baking pan, form into a loaf, and bake at 350° for 1 1/4 hours. For meatballs, mold into 1 1/2-inch balls, place on baking sheet, and bake at 350° for 20-30 minutes.

Ingredients

1 lb ground beef ◆ 1 cup S.V.P ◆ 3/4 cup tomato sauce ◆ 1/2 cup tomato paste ◆ 1 Tb onion powder ◆ 1 Tb garlic powder ◆ 1 tsp basil ◆ 1 tsp oregano ◆ salt ◆ pepper

GreySheet Cordon Bleu

Combine soy nuggets and bran and soy Parmesan with enough water to make a thick but pourable paste. Flatten each chicken breast by pounding with a mallet or the back of a knife; sprinkle each with spices. Place one slice ham and one slice soy cheese on each breast. Roll each chicken breast starting at narrow end. (If rolling is too awkward, fold them in half.) Place in an even layer in a baking dish and pour the soy mixture on top. Bake at 350° F for 30 minutes to an hour, or until chicken is done and soy is browned on top.

Ingredients

4 boneless, skinless chicken breasts ◆ 4 thin slices ham ◆ 4 thin slices soy cheese preferably provolone or mozzarella style ◆ ground oregano ◆ onion powder ◆ salt and pepper ◆ 1/2 cup combined soy nuggets and soy bran ◆ 1/4 cup soy parmesan (optional)

Grilled Salmon

Marinade a Salmon Steak about half an hour before grilling. Spray generously with Zero Calorie Butter Spray and grill over hot coals until fish flakes easily. (Approximately 8-10 min. depending on thickness). Weigh out serving.

Ingredients

2 tablespoons lemon juice ◆ 1 teaspoon dried Dill Weed ◆ 1 teaspoon Garlic and Herb Seasoning (I think McCormicks) ◆ Salt to taste

Island-Roasted Chicken

Preheat the oven to 375° F. Combine seasonings in a bowl and set aside. Brush the oil evenly over the chicken and inside the cavity. Insert the garlic slivers and the cloves under the skin. Sprinkle the seasoning mixture over the chikcen, under the skin, and inside the cavity. Stuff the thyme stems in the cavity and underneath the skin. Place the chicken on a rack in a roasting pan and roast for about 75 minutes, or until a leg can be easily twisted. Baste every 15 minutes with the pan juices.This works equally well with a breast of turkey.

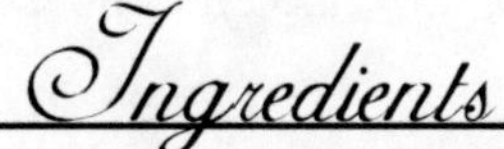

1 Tb olive oil ◆ 1 whole chicken washed and patted dry ◆ 6-8 cloves garlic slivered ◆ 1/2 Tb whole cloves ◆ 10-12 stems fresh thyme ◆ Seasonings: 1/2 tsp ground allspice ◆ 1/2 tsp ground nutmeg ◆ 1/2 tsp ground cloves ◆ 1/2 tsp ground cinnamon ◆ 1/2 tsp cayenne pepper ◆ 1/4 tsp (or more) salt

Jamaican Jerk Chicken

Place the hot pepper sauce in a shallow container. Add chicken, one piece at a time, turning to coat. Sprinkle salt, cinnamon and allspice over the chicken. Place the chicken, skin side up, in a single layer in a large shallow baking dish lined with foil. Bake at 400° F for 45 minutes or until the chicken is fork tender.

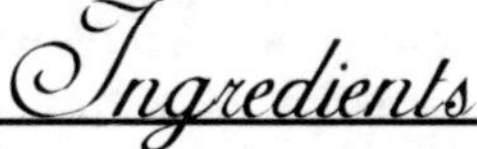

4 chicken quarters of the broiler/fryer type ◆ 1 tsp salt ◆ 1/2 tsp cinnamon ◆ 2 Tb hot pepper sauce (e.g. Tabasco) ◆ 1/2 tsp allspice

Keftadhes

Mix together all ingredients; shape into patties or meatballs. Place on baking sheet and bake in preheated 350° oven for about 30 minutes or until brown.

Ingredients

2 lbs ground meat ◆ 2 Tb onion soup mix ◆ 2 Tb parsley flakes ◆ 1 tsp chopped, bruised mint ◆ 1 tsp oregano

Kofta Curry

For koftas, fry onion powder, ginger, and garlic in 1 Tb oil until brown. (Or you may use ground ginger and garlic powder to mix with the meat.) Add to remaining kofta ingredients, mix well, and mold into balls 2 inches in diameter. For sauce, grind garlic and ginger to a paste in blender or food processor. Fry onion soup mix and garlic/ginger paste in remaining oil until light brown. Add tomato sauce, 3 cups water, salt, and cayenne. Bring to a boil. Add koftas and cook, uncovered, until all the water evaporates. Gently fold in garam masala.

Ingredients

Koftas sauce ◆ 1 lb ground beef ◆ 3 Tb onion soup mix ◆ 1 Tb onion powder ◆ 1 clove garlic ◆ 4 cloves garlic pressed ◆ 2 inches ginger peeled ◆ 1 inch ginger, grated ◆ 4 Tb tomato sauce ◆ salt to taste ◆ 2 tsp garam masala ◆ 1/4 tsp cayenne ◆ 1 Tb cayenne ◆ salt to taste ◆ 1 Tb vegetable oil

Koofteh Tabrizi

Mix all the meatball ingredients together and roll into balls, 2-1/2 inches in diameter, firmly packed. Refrigerate them for 1 hour. Heat the oil in a deep sauté pan and add the turmeric, tomato sauce, and salt. Stir for about 2 minutes, until sauce has absorbed oil. Add 2 cups water and bring to a boil. Take each herbed ball and roll it firmly; add the balls to the broth very carefully, one at a time, so that they do not fall apart. The water should just cover them. Cover the pan and cook over moderately low heat, without stirring, for 45 minutes. Check the thickness of the sauce; if it is too thin, remove lid, raise heat, and reduce to desired consistency. The meatballs may swell slightly as the soy granules absorb water.

Ingredients

Meatballs: 1 lb ground veal ◆ 1 1/2 cups soy granules ◆ 1/4 tsp pepper ◆ 2 Tb dried tarragon ◆ 2 bunches Italian flat-leaf parsley minced fine ◆ 1 Tb onion powder ◆ 1/2 cup chopped fresh dill
Sauce: 1 Tb oil ◆ 1/4 tsp turmeric ◆ 1 small can tomato sauce ◆ 1 tsp salt

Lamb Chop or Roast in Lemon Garlic Sauce

Combine lemon juice and grated garlic to make a sauce. Use sauce as a baste over the lamb and cook until done.

Ingredients

4 ozs lamb (chop or roast); lemon juice ◆ grated garlic

Lamb Chop(s)

Cook 1 lamb chop with seasonings to taste either in a dry frying pan or in a broiler.

Ingredients

lamb chop(s) with seasoning or salt and pepper

Lamb Vindaloo

Sightly roast the cumin seed and coriander seed by frying with no oil for a minute or so, stirring constantly. Grind these in a spice mill or coffee grinder and combine them into a paste with the other spices, the garlic, ginger, onion powder, tomato paste, and vinegar (not in the spice mill!). Combine the lamb and the spice in a large bowl or container and mix well. Refrigerate for 3-24 hours, mixing every few hours as convenient. (The marinating does add a lot of flavor and makes the meat much more tender, but if you are using a fairly tender cut of lamb, you can proceed directly from mixing to cooking.), When lamb has finished marinating, heat oil in a heavy-bottomed pan. Add lamb and spice paste and simmer over low heat for half an hour.

Ingredients

2 lbs cubed lamb ◆ 1 Tb coriander seed ◆ 1/2 Tb cumin seed ◆ 3 Tb tomato paste ◆ 14 cloves garlic pressed ◆ 6 bay leaves ◆ 2-inch piece fresh ginger peeled and grated or finely chopped ◆ 1/2 tsp ground black pepper ◆ 1/2 tsp cardamon seed ◆ 1/2 tsp cinnamon ◆ 1/2 tsp cloves ◆ 1/2 tsp cayenne ◆ 1 tsp ground mustard seed ◆ 1 tsp turmeric ◆ 1 Tb onion powder ◆ 3 Tb cider vinegar ◆ 1 Tb olive oil

Lavender and Thyme Roasted Poussins

Line a roasting pan with thick foil and preheat the oven to about 475° F/ 250° C. Remove gizzards from chicken or poussins and trim away excess fat. Rinse clean in warm water. Arrange breast-up in the pan. Using the tip of a small sharp knife and your fingers, carefully separate the skin above the breast from the meat, being careful not to tear the skin. Whisk remaining ingredients together in a bowl. Pour approximately half this mixture under the skin of the bird(s), and the remainder into the cavity. Pin or tie the legs and tails to seal the cavity. Roast for 30-60 minutes, depending on the size of the birds. The skin should be brown and crackly. An instant-read thermometer inserted into the thickest part of the thigh should read 170°F.

Ingredients

1 small roasting chicken or 2 poussins/Cornish hens ◆ 2 tsp dried untreated lavender flowers ◆ 1 tsp thyme leaves ◆ 2 Tb lemon juice ◆ 1 Tb balsamic vinegar ◆ 1 Tb light olive oil ◆ salt and pepper

Lavender Cream Chicken

Cut chicken into bite-sized pieces. Heat oil in large deep frying pan and brown chicken lightly on all sides. Reduce heat to medium and add garlic, herbs, and vinegar to deglaze the pan. When vinegar has evaporated, add the soy cream cheese, salt and pepper, and water or soymilk. Stir until the soy cream cheese dissolves into a smooth sauce. Reduce heat to very low and simmer for about 15 minutes or until sauce clings solidly to chicken

Ingredients

1 lb boneless chicken ◆ 1 Tb olive oil ◆ 2 cloves garlic, chopped ◆ 1 tsp combination marjoram/thyme/summer savory/basil/rosemary/fennel seeds ◆ 1 tsp lavender flowers ◆ 2 Tb white vinegar ◆ ½ cup soy cream cheese ◆ 1 cup soy milk or water ◆ salt and pepper

Lemongrass Meatballs

Combine seasonings in a small bowl. Place ground meat in a large bowl, pour seasonings over it, and combine thoroughly. Cover and refrigerate for several hours or overnight. Preheat oven to 350°. Form marinated meat into 1-2 inch diameter meatballs and place on a foil-covered baking sheet. Bake for approximately 30 minutes.

Ingredients

2 Tb soy sauce ◆ 1 Tb white vinegar ◆ 2 1/2 Tb fresh or 1 Tb dried lemon grass ◆ 1 Tb peanut oil (optional) ◆ 2 cloves garlic pressed or 1 Tb garlic powder ◆ 1 tsp red pepper flakes ◆ 1/4 cup fresh or 1 Tb dried mint leaves ◆ 1 tsp liquid sweetener ◆ 1 lb ground beef (or other ground meat)

Lemongrass-Grilled Beef

Combine soy sauce, oil, vinegar, lemongrass, garlic, red pepper flakes, mint leaves, and sweetener in a blender or food-processor and purée the hell out of them. Transfer into a shallow baking dish. Thread the beef onto skewers and add to the marinade. Refrigerate at least 2-4 hours, turning once. Preheat the grill or broiler, very hot. Grill skewers for 2 to 3 minutes on each side.

Ingredients

2 Tb soy sauce ◆ 1 Tb white vinegar ◆ 2 1/2 Tb minced fresh lemongrass ◆ 1 Tb peanut oil ◆ 2 cloves garlic pressed ◆ 1 tsp red pepper flakes ◆ 1/4 cup fresh mint leaves ◆ 1 tsp liquid sweetener ◆ 1 1/2 lbs beef, sliced into thin strips

Lemon-Ricotta Pancakes

Separate egg carefully, white into one bowl, yolk in the other. To the yolk add lemon juice, sweetener, ground texturized soy protein, and ricotta and whisk thoroughly to combine. Beat egg white with salt until it forms stiff peaks using a hand-mixer. Whisk about 1/4 of the egg white into the yolk mixture, then gently fold in the rest. You should have a fluffy yellow mass rather like an uncooked soufflé. Heavily spray a skillet with Pam, and heat over medium-high heat. When hot, pile the batter into the pan (makes two large or 3 small pancakes) and cook for 2-3 minutes per side. The pancakes will remain thick and fluffy, so be careful not to burn them, for fear of having them be undercooked.

Ingredients

1 egg ◆ 1 1/2 ounces ricotta cheese ◆ 1/2 ounce ground texturized soy protein ◆ 1 tablespoon lemon juice ◆ sweetener ◆ salt

Louisiana Roast Beef

Combine onion soup mix and seasonings in a small bowl with 2 Tb water; mix well. Place the roast in a large roasting pan, fat side up. With a large knife make 6-12 deep slits in the meat, down to a depth of about 1/2 inch from the bottom; do not cut all the way through. Fill the pockets with the seasoning mixture, reserving 1 Tb to rup over the top of the roast. Bake uncovered at 300° until a meat thermometer reads 160° for medium doneness, about 3 hours.

Ingredients

2 Tb onion powder ◆ 1 tsp salt ◆ 1 tsp white pepper ◆ 3/4 tsp black pepper ◆ 3/4 tsp minced garlic ◆ 1/2 tsp dry mustard ◆ 1/2 tsp cayenne ◆ 1 (3 1/2-4 lb) boneless sirloin roast or top round roast

Lucanian Meatballs

Preheat oven to 350 °. Combine ingredients thoroughly in a large mixing bowl. Mold into small meatballs and place on foil-lined baking sheet. Bake for about 30 minutes.

Ingredients

1/2 tsp pepper ◆ 1/2 tsp cumin ◆ 1 tsp savory ◆ 1 Tb parsley ◆ pinch of rosemary ◆ 1/4 tsp ground cloves ◆ 1 lb ground meat

Mayan Chicken

Combine everything except the chicken and whisk until well mixed. Add chicken and coat thoroughly. Cover and chill 2-4 hours or overnight. Stir once in a while. Grill over medium to hot oiled grill 5-7 min on each side until chicken is white in the center. Fairly hot and pleasantly tangy. Reduce the quantity of chipotle purée if you need to.

Ingredients

3-4 garlic cloves, chopped ◆ 2 Tb chipotle purée ◆ 2 Tb fresh cilantro chopped ◆ 2 Tb achiote (annato) oil (or mix vegetable oil with 1 tsp paprika) ◆ 1 Tb balsamic vinegar ◆ 2 kaffir lime leaves, boiled and soaked ◆ 2 tsp ground cumin ◆ 2 tsp dried oregano ◆ 1/2 tsp salt ◆ 1/2 tsp fresh ground pepper ◆ 1 1/2 lb boneless skinless chicken breasts cut in wide strips

Meat with Whole Spices

Heat oil in a heavy-bottomed pan over medium heat. When it is very hot, put the spices in quickly in this order: first the cinnamon, then the black peppercorns, cloves, cardamom pods, and bay leaves, and finally the hot pepper. When the pepper begins to change color and darken, add the pieces of meat and the salt. Stir for 5 minutes or until the pot begins to make boiling noises. Cover, lower heat, and cook for approximately 1 hour or until the meat is tender. Remove the cover and continue cooking for a final 3 to 5 minutes, gently stirring the meat pieces. Sprinkle garam masala over the top before serving.

Ingredients

1 Tb vegetable oil ◆ 1 stick cinnamon ◆ 20 whole black peppercorns ◆ 15 whole cloves ◆ 10 whole cardamom pods ◆ 2 bay leave ◆ 1 whole dried hot red pepper ◆ 2 lbs boneless beef (or lamb) cubed ◆ 1-1 1/2 tsp salt ◆ 1 tsp garam masala

Mexican-Style Chicken

Poach chicken pieces until almost tender, about 15 minutes, in 1 quart of well-seasoned water, adding bay leaf, 2 garlic cloves, peppercorns, and salt. Let chicken cool in broth. Measure the oil into a baking dish and lay the chicken on top of it. Combine tomato paste, jalapeño powder, salt, black pepper, onion powder, and oregano with 2 cups reserved chicken stock. Boil 5 minutes and add the remaining garlic. Pour all of the sauce over the chicken, cover, and bake in 350° oven for 15 minutes, until bubbly.

Ingredients

2 lbs chicken pieces ◆ 1quart water ◆ 1 bay leaf ◆ 2 cloves garlic, peeled and flattened, a few whole black peppercorns ◆ 1 Tb salt ◆ 1 Tb onion powder ◆ 3 Tb olive oil ◆ 2 Tb tomato paste ◆ 1 tsp jalapeño powder ◆ 1/2 tsp oregano ◆ 4 cloves garlic pressed

Milk Chocolate Quake

Freeze milk in an ice cube tray Combine the frozen milk and diet soda and mix in a blender. The same shake can be made with other diet sodas. If you prefer not to freeze your milk, you can blend using ice cubes.

Ingredients

1 cup whole milk ◆ 1 can Canfield's diet chocolate soda

Moroccan Meatballs

Mix meat with all seasonings and pound or knead vigorously until very smooth and pasty. Shape small lumps of the mixture around skewers. Grill, or bake on foil-covered tray, less the skewers.

Ingredients

2 lbs finely ground beef ◆ 2 Tb onion powder ◆ 3 Tb parsley flakes ◆ 1/2 tsp marjoram ◆ 1/4 tsp ground cumin ◆ 1/4 tsp ground coriander ◆ 1/2 tsp Harissa, salt and black pepper, 1/4 tsp cayenne

Neua Pad Prik (Beef Chile)

Combine beef slices, sweetener, ginger, garlic and soy in a glass or ceramic bowl. Mix well and marinate 1 hour or longer. Heat oil in a wok. Drain beef; set marinade aside. Stir-fry beef in oil until done. Add marinade and beef stock. Reduce heat, cook 3 minutes, stir in soy flour roux.

Ingredients

1 pound lean beef, cut into thin strips ◆ 1 x 2 inches, a one-inch chunk of ginger peeled and minced ◆ 2 cloves garlic minced ◆ 1 tsp liquid sweetener ◆ 3 Tb soy sauce ◆ 1 Tb canola or peanut oil ◆ 4 Serrano or 8 "bird" (Thai) peppers soaked and sliced ◆ 1 Tb soy flour mixed with 2 Tb water

Neua Pad Prik (Beef Chile)

Combine beef slices, sweetener, ginger, garlic and soy in a glass or ceramic bowl. Mix well and marinate 1 hour or longer. Heat oil in a wok. Drain beef; set marinade aside. Stir-fry beef in oil until done. Add marinade and beef stock. Reduce heat, cook 3 minutes, stir in soy flour roux.

Ingredients

1 pound lean beef, cut into thin strips ◆ 1 x 2 inches, a one-inch chunk of ginger peeled and minced ◆ 2 cloves garlic minced ◆ 1 tsp liquid sweetener ◆ 3 Tb soy sauce ◆ 2 Tb canola or peanut oil ◆ 4 Serrano or 8 "bird" (Thai) peppers soaked and sliced ◆ 1 Tb soy flour mixed with 2 Tb water

Omelet

Cook egg in small, round pan to form round shape. Once egg is cooked, Add ham or cheese on top. Top with tomato sauce and spices. Fold egg to form omelet shape. Microwave for a few seconds, if desired, to melt cheese.

Ingredients

1 egg ◆ 1 ounce cheddar soy cheese or 1/2 ounce regular cheddar cheese or 2 ounces bacon or ham ◆ 1 tablespoon tomato sauce ◆ pinch of garlic/cilantro or chili pepper

One Pot Cassoulet

Brown the chicken thighs and sausages in the oil over high heat. Add the pancetta to the frying pan and fry until brown. Reduce heat and add 3/4 of the garlic; cook for a minute more. Use the vinegar to deglaze the frying pan. Pour 1 cup water into the pan along with the onion powder, tomato paste, sweetener, bay leaf, rosemary, and half the parsley. Add the soybeans, season with salt and pepper, and bring to a boil. Simmer very gently, half-covered, for about 40 minutes, stirring occasionally. Add the soy nuts and remaining garlic and parsley. Stir to mix well and allow to heat through.

Ingredients

6 boneless chicken thighs or 1 lb diced chicken or turkey thigh meat ◆ 1 Tb olive oil ◆ 6 all-beef sausages sliced into rounds ◆ 2 strips bacon or pancetta shredded ◆ 4 cloves garlic pressed ◆ 2 Tb balsamic vinegar ◆ 1 Tb onion powder ◆ 1 Tb tomato paste ◆ 1 tsp liquid sweetener ◆ 1 bay leaf ◆ 1 sprig fresh rosemary ◆ 4 Tb chopped parsley ◆ 2 cans white soybeans, drained and rinsed ◆ 1 cup soy nuts, salt and pepper

Pancakes

Combine ingredients in blender and mix until you have smooth batter. Preheat flat pan and coat with non-stick spray. Pour batter, cook until light brown and turn and finish cooking on other side. Should resemble real pancake.

Ingredients

1 egg ◆ 2 oz. Farmers cheese ◆ sweetener to taste ◆ dash of salt

Party Mix

Combine TVP, soy granules, and soy nuts in a large bowl. Then add Worcestershire, soy sauce to flavor and moisten just a bit, add salt, pepper, and Cajun spices to taste. Mix all together well using hands. Spread out in thin layer on a cookie sheet. Bake at 350 degrees for 30 minutes, stirring several times and re-spreading. Then let air-dry until cool. Weigh 4 oz. of the mix into sealtight baggies or store in Tupperware and weigh out when needed.

Ingredients

TVP ◆ soy granules ◆ dry roasted soynuts ◆ worcestershire ◆ soy sauce ◆ salt ◆ pepper ◆ Cajun spices

Perfect Roast Chicken

Trim the fat from the bird and remove giblets. Slip two peeled garlic cloves and a sprig of fresh marjoram (you can use any herb - except rosemary) under the skin of the breast on each side. Generously sprinkle kosher salt and pepper all over the bird, being particularly liberal with the salt. Refrigerate overnight or for 24 hours. Place the chicken on a pan (you can use a rack if you like so the juices fall down into the pan) and cook it for approximately 25 - 40 minutes depending on the oven temperature. The oven temperature should be as hot as you can get it -- maybe 450 - 500 degrees. When the juices run clear and the chicken is brown, it is done. The important thing is to keep an eye on the chicken so it doesn't overcook. Let the chicken sit for awhile (5 min.), cut it up and Enjoy!!! Note: This recipe works equally well for a cut-up chicken or several chicken breasts.

Ingredients

1 whole chicken about 3 lbs ◆ 2 cloves garlic peeled ◆ sprig fresh marjoram ◆ kosher salt ◆ pepper

Persian Ground Lamb

Heat oil in a large skillet. Add the ground lamb and cook until browned and crumbly. Drain off fat, if necessary. Add onion powder, allspice, curry powder, salt and pepper, and 2 Tb water to cooked meat. Cook 3 minutes to blend flavors. Add soy nuts, reduce heat and cover. Simmer over low heat 15 minutes, stirring to prevent sticking.

Ingredients

1 Tb almond oil ◆ 1 Tb onion powder ◆ 1 1/2 lbs ground lamb ◆ 1/4 tsp ground allspice ◆ 1/4 tsp Madras curry powder ◆ Salt and pepper to taste ◆ 1/2 cup soy nuts

Pizza Recipe

Start by weighing 4 ounces equivalent of tofu flat and mozzarella cheese, and well done, blotted, sausage or other protein topping. Cover the flat with layers of 1 oz tomato sauce, then mozzarella, then other toppings, the another 1 oz. of tomato sauce. Put the whole flat on a skillet over med. heat until the cheese melts. The tofu cooks more (and gets more crispy and tender) as it cooks on the skillet.

Ingredients

4 ounce equivalent of Tofu flats, available in Oriental groceries ◆ 4 ounces mozzarella cheese, well done, blotted, sausage or other protein topping ◆ 2 oz tomato sauce

Pollo al Ajillo

Sprinkle the chicken with salt. Heat the oil in a shallow flameproof casserole and brown the chicken on all sides over medium-high heat. Add the chopped garlic, reduce heat to medium, and cook, stirring occasionally, for 30 minutes. Stir in the minced garlic, parsley, and vinegar. Cover and cook for 15 minutes more.

Ingredients

2 lbs chicken meat, cut into small serving pieces ◆ salt ◆ 1 Tb olive oil ◆ 6 cloves garlic, coarsely chopped ◆ 1 clove garlic, pressed ◆ 1 Tb minced parsley ◆ 2 Tb white vinegar

Ranch Chicken Chipotle

Place chicken in a pot with the water, the 8 whole garlic cloves, and the salt. Simmer for 30 to 40 minutes, until very tender. Remove from pan and allow to cool. Pull the meat from the bones and tear into pieces. Save 1/2 cup of the liquid from cooking the chicken. Heat olive oil in a large skillet and add minced garlic. Add tomato paste, chipotle purée, and chicken stock. Mix thoroughly and allow to come to a boil. Add the shredded chicken and the cilantro and simmer for 15-20 minutes. Sauce should be fairly thick.

Ingredients

2 bone-in chicken breasts ◆ 2 quarts of water ◆ 1 Tb onion powder ◆ 1 Tb salt ◆ 11 cloves of garlic (8 whole, 3 minced) ◆ 2 Tb tomato paste ◆ 2 Tb chipotle purée ◆ 2 tsp minced cilantro

Ribs

Buy rack of ribs in the grocery store cut them so they fit in a crockpot. Add about 3/4 bottle of Texas best original recipe. Set on low and let slow cook overnight (or about 8 hrs). The meat will fall off the bone and you can weigh it after cooked.

Ingredients

Rack of ribs ◆ Texas Best "original recipe" BBQ sauce

Roast Duck w/Soy Sauce and Chinese 5 Spice Powder

After removing and discarding the packet of orange sauce that comes packed inside with the giblets, liver, and heart and rinsing the duck well both inside and out I dry it carefully with paper towels and put it into a large rectangular glass oven dish (if you use one large enough you won't have to turn the duck at all during cooking). To season the duck ahead of time I use abstinent soy sauce (check with sponsor as to what you can use -- I have a huge, ancient bottle I'm told is no longer made--it's Eden brand wheat, sugar, and alcohol free). I smear this all over the duck, inside and out (be sure to get under the wings). Then I take Chinese 5 Spice Powder and sprinkle all over the duck and rub it in.After that I just follow the instructions on the wrapper the duck came in. I love this much better than the duck in Chinese restaurants, because they always remove some of the fat. I actually have to work hard to get myself to weigh in any of the duck meat as long as there's any skin left. Be careful because it can make you queasy if you're not a hardened grease addict!

Ingredients

Fresh or Frozen Duck ◆ Abstinent Soy Sauce ◆ Chinese 5 Spice Powder

Roasted Chicken with Rosemary, Lemon, Soy Sauce

Remove and discard giblets and neck from chicken. Rinse chicken under cold running water; drain well and pat dry. Place chicken breast side up, on rack in shallow roasting pan. Blend soy sauce, lemon juice, rosemary, and garlic. Spray zero-calorie butter spray on top of spice mixture and on chicken. Brush chicken cavity and skin thoroughly with mixture. Roast at 350 for 1 hour and 45 minutes, or until meat thermometer inserted into thickest part of thigh registers 185, brushing with soy mixture every 30 minutes. Remove chicken from oven and let stand 10 minutes before carving. Weigh 4 ounces and serve.

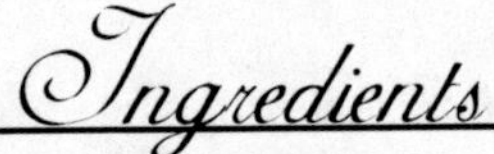

4 pounds whole chicken ◆ 3 tablespoons soy sauce, daily allowance fresh lemon juice ◆ zero-calorie butter spray (olive flavor is good) ◆ 2 teaspoons dried rosemary or fresh rosemary, crumbled ◆ 2 cloves garlic, pressed

Roman Meatballs

Combine all ingredients except olive oil and mix thoroughly. Form into 20 balls and pan-brown in the olive oil. (Do this in 2 or 3 batches.) Bake at 350° for about 30 minutes.

Ingredients

2 lbs lean ground beef ◆ 1/2 lb ground pork ◆ 6 oz pancetta or bacon diced very small ◆ 6 oz prosciutto sliced thin and chopped ◆ 2 Tb parsley flakes ◆ 3 cloves garlic pressed ◆ salt and freshly ground black pepper to taste ◆ 1 Tb olive oil for browning

Sashimi

Serve separately.

Ingredients

4 oz. Sashimi (raw tuna, salmon, yellowtail) ◆ 1 tablespoon ginger dressing ◆ 1/2 cup boiled cold carrots ◆ 1 cup salad with tomato and cucumber ◆ Sashimi condiments: Wasabi (horseradish mustard)

Scone

Mix together soy flour and milk. Add the soynuts and flavoring. Add sweetener to taste. Spray the bottom of a small pyrex or tupperware dish with Pam and spoon in the mixture to make like a big "scone." Microwave for 5 to 6 minutes. Cool and turn out.

Ingredients

2 oz. soyflour ◆ 4 oz. milk ◆ 1/2 oz. soynuts ◆ 1 teaspoon alcohol free vanilla or maple flavoring ◆ 1 dropper full of alcohol free stevia or other sweetener

Sesame Sauce

Blend until smooth.

Ingredients

1/3 cup rice vinegar ◆ 3.5 oz. soy butter ◆ 2/3 cup hot water ◆ 2 tablespoons reduced sodium soy sauce ◆ 4 cloves garlic ◆ 1 package Equal or Sweet N Low ◆ 1 teaspoon crushed red pepper flakes

Shake and Bake Chicken

Put all the ingredients, except the chicken, in a sturdy plastic bag. Shake to mix. Drop chicken pieces one or two at a time into bag and shake to coat. Place coated chicken pieces in a pan sprayed baking dish. Bake at 325 for 60 to 90 minutes.

Ingredients

1 cup Soy flour ◆ 3 teaspoons Paprika ◆ 1 teaspoon Poultry seasoning ◆ 1 teaspoon Sage ◆ 1 teaspoon Thyme ◆ 1 teaspoon Salt ◆ 1 teaspoon Pepper ◆ 1 chicken cut in to parts (i.e. leg, thigh, breast, etc.)

Shrimp, Boiled

Bring water to a boil, with crab boil and salt added. Add shrimp. Return to a boil and cook 3 to 4 minutes. Remove from water at once. Measure 4 oz. and serve hot or chilled. Do not overcook or undersalt! Shrimp may be shelled and deveined before cooking, if preferred.

Ingredients

1 to 4 pounds shrimp ◆ 1 bag abstinent crab boil, seasoning salt

Shredded Chicken Yucatan

Place the peppercorns, oregano, and salt in a spice or coffee grinder and grind to a powder. Combine this powder with the onion powder, the first two cloves garlic and the vinegar and make a paste. Set aside. Roast both heads of garlic in a 350° oven for 20 minutes and allow to cool. (Be sure they are truly cooked to liquid mushiness, or there will be a harsh taste to your chicken.) Place the chicken in a stockpot with water to cover, dried habañero, salt, and oregano, and simmer until the chicken is tender, about 30 minutes. Drain the chicken, reserving the broth, and transfer it to an oven-proof dish. Add the peppercorn paste and bake uncovered at 350° until golden brown, about 30 minutes. Peel the roasted garlic and combine it with the reserved chicken stock. Add the chiles and simmer for 5 minutes. Add the kaffir lime leaves, bring to a boil, and remove from heat immediately. When cool, purée in a blender.Skin the chicken and shred the meat from the bones. Add the purée to the chicken and mix well. Heat through. This dish should be thick but not soupy.

Ingredients

10 peppercorns ◆ 1/4 tsp ground oregano ◆ 1/2 tsp salt ◆ 2 cloves garlic, pressed ◆ 1 Tb vinegar ◆ 1 Tb onion powder ◆ 2 whole heads garlic ◆ 2 kaffir lime leaves soaked ◆ 3 lbs chicken thighs ◆ 1 tsp salt ◆ 1/2 tsp ground oregano 1 dried habañero chile

Shrimp, Boiled

Bring water to a boil, with crab boil and salt added. Add shrimp. Return to a boil and cook 3 to 4 minutes. Remove from water at once. Measure 4 oz. and serve hot or chilled. Do not overcook or undersalt! Shrimp may be shelled and deveined before cooking, if preferred.

Ingredients

1 to 4 pounds shrimp ◆ 1 bag abstinent crab boil ◆ seasoning salt

Shrimp, Stir Fried

If shrimp are purchased frozen, thaw out. Pat shrimp dry with paper towels, squeezing out water weight. Spray non-stick skillet with Pam over high heat. Add shrimp and cook, stirring briskly, for 3 minutes, just until shrimp are pink and cooked through. Do not overcook shrimp, it toughens them. Weigh 4 oz. and serve. This tastes great cold over salad!

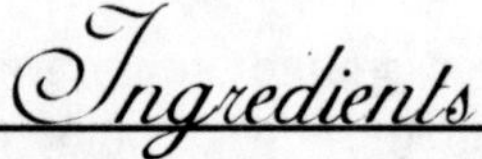

1 pound small fresh-frozen shrimp, cooked, peeled, deveined ◆ zero-calorie butter spray ◆ abstinent seasoned salt

Sindhi Meat

After the meat has marinated, pour contents of the bowl into a wide 4-quart cooking pot. Add the fennel and onion seeds. Bring to a boil. Cover, lower heat, and simmer about 1 hour. Lift off cover, raise heat, and boil rapidly until most of the liquid evaporates. Now add the oil and keep stirring and frying over a medium flame. A thickish sauce should cling to the meat, which browns as the liquid cooks down.

Ingredients

2 1/2 lbs cubed beef ◆ 2 Tb onion powder, a piece of fresh ginger,2 inches long and 1 inch wide coarsely chopped ◆ 6 cloves garlic pressed ◆ 1 Tb ground coriander ◆ 2 tsp ground cumin ◆ 1 tsp ground turmeric ◆ 1/8- 1/2 tsp cayenne ◆ 3 Tb cider vinegar (optional) ◆ 1 tsp salt ◆ 2 tsp whole fennel seeds ◆ 1 tsp whole black onion seeds (kalonji) ◆ 1 Tb vegetable oil

Southern Fried Chicken

Whip eggs and red hot together, place raw chicken in eggs, use right away or let sit for 3 hours in the fridge. When ready to cook, mix soy flour, garlic powder, salt, pepper, paprika, and any other desired spice in a dish. Heat about 1/2 inch to 1 inch of oil in a fry pan.Take chicken from egg mix and coat in soy flour mix. Measure and serve.

Ingredients

2 lbs. skinless, boneless chicken pieces ◆ 4 eggs ◆ Frank's Red Hot Sauce ◆ soy flour ◆ garlic powder ◆ salt ◆ pepper ◆ paprika

Smothered Chicken

To butterfly a chicken, take a large, heavy cleaver and deliver a mighty blow parallel to the spine. Wrench chicken open and flatten it a bit. Use a hammer if you have to. If this is all too violent for you, have the butcher do it. Otherwise this is a great recipe for really frustrating days. Sprinkle salt and pepper on both sides of the chicken. Fold the wings underneath. Secure the wings in place. Heat the oil in a heavy, cast iron skillet large enough to hold the flattened chicken comfortably. Put the chicken in the skillet, skin side down. Cover the chicken with a plate, put about 5 pounds of weight on top of the plate, and cook over low heat until the skin is nicely browned (about 25 minutes). Remove weight and plate and turn the chicken skin side up. Replace the plate and weight and cook for another 15 minutes. Remove the chicken from the skillet. Pour off the fat, reserving the amount indicated in the ingredients. Whisk the soy flour into the fat. Gradually add the water. Cook, whisking steadily, until thickened. Add more water if you need to. Return the chicken, skin side up, to the pan; add salt and pepper to taste. Replace the plate and the weight. Cook over low heat until the chicken is exceptionally tender (about 30 minutes). Turn off heat. Remove the chicken and dismember thoroughly, clawing the meat from the bones (I told you this was an aggressive recipe). Return meat to the pan and cook together with the gravy until everything is heated through and bubbling nicely. Very tasty results. Measure and serve.

Ingredients

1 chicken ◆ about 3 1/2 lbs butterflied (split down the backbone) ◆ 2 Tb soy flour ◆ 1 1/2 cups water ◆ 2 Tb fat from cooking the chicken (see the instructions) ◆ Salt ◆ Pepper ◆ 2 Tb olive oil

Soy Croutons

After measuring soy, coat with zero-calorie butter spray.

Ingredients

1 ounce texturized soy protein chunks zero-calorie butter spray (i.e. Oriental, Garlic...)

Soy Milk, How To Make

Rinse and soak the beans overnight (or at least 10 hours) in the fridge. When ready, drain and rinse the beans. Either grind the beans into a paste using a grain mill and add to a pot of 12 cups boiling water OR process the beans in a blender or food processor with boiling water (3/4 cup beans to 1 3/4 cup boiling water at a time) and pour into a big heavy pot. (Note: It is important to not over estimate your blenders abilities. Be careful to not burn out your blender while grinding beans. A food processor offers better results (with sharp blade)). Bring this mixture to a boil while stirring over medium to high heat. Turn down immediately after it starts to boil, or you'll have a mess. Now let it simmer (no stirring necessary) for 20-30 minutes. Meanwhile... line a colander with a thin cloth, and set it up over a big bowl or another pot. When the soymilk is cooked, ladle it into the colander, straining the pulp (called okara) in the cloth and allowing the milk to collect in the bowl. Make sure to squeeze all the milk you can from the okara before transferring it into a jug or two to cool. You may add more water, sweetener, vanilla extract, or sea salt. The okara can be steamed for an hour and used as a soy protein, too, like tofu patties. Measure soy protein or soy milk as 4 ounces. Makes a gallon or so. Preparation time is 1/2 - 1 hour.

Ingredients

2 cups of dried soy beans, water

Soy Muffin

Combine the soy with the spices and sweetener in a small bowl. Add 3-4 Tbl. of diet soda or carbonated water, stir, and leave mixture to expand. When soy is puffy and fairly solid, scrape into a baking cup, and place in a muffin pan. Bake for approximately 30 minutes at 350°F. The resulting muffin is 1 oz. of protein. Serving ideas: heat and sprinkle with cinnamon, sweetener, and zero calorie butter spray. These are good to travel with and quite filling!

Ingredients

Per Muffin: 1 ounce combined finely ground texturized soy protein and coarsely ground texturized soy protein ◆ 3 tablespoons diet lemon/lime soda (7 Up, Sprite) or carbonated water ◆ sweetener to taste (I use 6 Equal packets) ◆ 1/4 teaspoon each: cinnamon ◆ nutmeg ◆ allspice ◆ ginger ◆ and salt ◆ paper baking cups

Soy Nut Crunch

Measure soy nuts in small, shallow plastic or glass container. Spray with zero-calorie butter spray. Top with sweetener and seasoned salt. Microwave for 30 seconds, or until sticky.

Ingredients

1 ounce dry, halved ◆ unroasted soy nuts ◆ zero-calorie spray butter ◆ sweetener ◆ abstinent seasoned salt

Soy Pancakes

Beat egg in a large bowl and add reconstituted texturized soy protein, sweetener and cinnamon. Continue to mix until smooth. Spray Pam in a non-stick skillet over medium flame. Recipe makes 2 medium-sized pancakes; the smaller they are, the easier they are to turn. Cook like regular pancakes. Top with sweetener, cinnamon, and zero calorie butter spray. Makes 3/4 portion of a protein, as written. You may also add fruit to the batter after it has been mixed.

Ingredients

1 egg ◆ 1 ounce ground texturized soy protein, reconstituted with 1 tablespoon vanilla ◆ 4 packets sweetener ◆ 1 teaspoon cinnamon

Soy Pizza, Small Crust

Preheat oven to 425° F. Brush the oil over a baking sheet or pizza pan. Mix texturized soy protein, salt, and about 2 Tbl. water in a bowl, and combine to form dough. Roll between sheets of non-stick baking paper until you have a flat crust, or spread with your fingers onto a baking sheet. Spread the tomato sauce on top with a brush or spatula. Sprinkle the pepperoni and soy cheese on top. Bake for 10-15 minutes.

Ingredients

2 ounces finely ground texturized soy protein ◆ 1 ounce pepperoni ◆ 1 ounce grated mozzarella soy cheese ◆ 1 teaspoon salt ◆ 2 ounces tomato paste/sauce mixed with Italian seasoning (or diet catsup may be substituted)

Soy Tortilla with Soy Nut Butter

Combine first 3 ingredients. Flatten like tortilla on baking sheet (keep hands damp or flour mixture sticks to them). Cook in 350 degree oven for 15 minutes. Spread with 1-ounce soy nut butter.

Ingredients

3 oz. soy flour ◆ Club soda or plain water ◆ salt ◆ 1 oz. soy nut butter

Soya con Pollo

Combine turmeric, saffron, salt, 1 Tb oil and about 2 Tb warm water in a sealable container and whisk together to form marinade. Add the chicken meat and mix thoroughly with the marinade. Seal the container and refrigerate at least 30 minutes. Heat the remaining 2 Tb oil in a large, heavy skillet, preferably non-stick. Remove chicken from marinade, reserving the marinade, and brown in the oil. Remove from pan. Add the soy nuggets or granules, the onion powder, and the garlic powder. Stir-fry until soy is toasted. Add 1-2 cups water, the oregano, pepper, and paprika. Bring to a boil, then reduce heat to low. Add the reserved marinade, the tomato paste, chili pepper, and parsley. Mix thoroughly. Add the chicken pieces, cover, and cook over low heat 30 minutes or until chicken is done.

Ingredients

1-2 lbs chicken meat, cut into bite-sized pieces ◆ 1/4 tsp turmeric ◆ 1/8 tsp saffron threads crushed ◆ 1 Tb lemon juice ◆ 1/4 tsp salt ◆ 1 Tb vegetable oil ◆ 1 cup soy nuggets or granules ◆ 1 Tb onion powder ◆ 1 Tb garlic powder ◆ 1/2 tsp oregano ◆ 1/4 tsp ground black pepper ◆ 1/4 tsp paprika ◆ 2 Tb tomato paste ◆ 1/2 tsp red pepper flakes ◆ 2 Tb minced fresh parsley

Soybeans, Cooked

Soak your soybeans in water overnight. Add enough water to cover them about an inch. You may need to add more throughout cooking if a lot evaporates. Add desired amount of soy sauce (and salt if you want). Add enough to make the cooking water a light brown color. Cook them mostly covered (put the lid on the pan loose, so steam can escape) on a stove at medium heat until tender. (There should actually be a very slight crunch when they are done). A 14-ounce bag of dried soybeans takes a little over an hour.

Ingredients

dried soy beans (check your local Asian supermarket) ◆ soy sauce ◆ salt (optional)

Soyburgers

Mash cooked black soybeans, then add and mix all ingredients except for oil. Let mixture sit for a few minutes then divide into 2 or 3 burgers. Heat oil in frying pan and add burgers. Brown on both sides. Freeze after cooking for later use.

Ingredients

1 egg ◆ 2 oz. cooked black soybeans ◆ 1/8 cup wheat germ ◆ 1 teaspoon dehydrated onion flakes ◆ 1 teaspoon prepared mustard ◆ one tablespoon soy sauce or Worcestershire sauce ◆ 1/2 teaspoon garlic powder ◆ 1 tablespoon oil

Spicy Grilled Chicken

Combine all ingredients except chicken in a large sealable container. Add the chicken pieces and marinate for one hour at room temperature, turning or shaking occasionally. When the chicken is done marinating and the grill is ready, remove chicken from container and broil about 30 minutes. Reserve marinade and use it to baste chicken while it's grilling.

Ingredients

2-4 lbs chicken, 3 Tb vegetable oil ◆ 2 Tb lemon juice ◆ 2 cloves garlic pressed ◆ 1 1/2 tsp finely chopped fresh oregano (or 1/2 tsp dried) ◆ 1 tsp salt ◆ 1/4 tsp crushed dried red chilies ◆ 1/4 tsp pepper

Spicy Thai Style Ground Chicken with Basil

Heat oil in wok on high. Add chicken and stir fry 45 sec. Add garlic and hot pepper flakes. Cook until the chicken is no longer pink, about 2-3 minutes. Add onion powder, lemon juice, soy sauce, and sweetener. Stir-fry 30 seconds. Add basil immediately before removing from heat and stir until it is just wilted

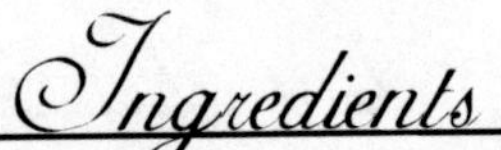

1 Tb vegetable oil ◆ 1 Tb hot oil ◆ 12 oz ground chicken, turkey, or beef ◆ 1 Tb onion powder ◆ 1 Tb lemon juice ◆ 2 cloves garlic, minced ◆ 1/2 tsp red pepper flakes ◆ 2 Tb soy sauce ◆ 1 tsp liquid sweetener ◆ 1/2 c fresh basil leaves chopped

Strawberries and Pineapple Tropical Delight

Measure and combine all fruit and protein in food processor. Blend until mixed well. Pour into shallow plastic dish with cover. Place in freezer for at least 4 hours. Top with coffee syrup, or extract, and sweetener. If frozen solid, place in microwave for 30 seconds, to thaw, before serving.

Ingredients

1/2 cup cottage cheese or 1 cup yogurt ◆ 1 cup mixed pineapple and strawberries ◆ sweetener ◆ sugar-free Da Vinci Coconut coffee syrup or Frontier Coconut extract

Thai Turkey Burgers

In a small dish combine the garlic, ginger, cilantro, mint, basil, lemon juice, soy sauce, sesame oil and sweetener and mix well. Add the turkey and soy nuggets and mix lightly, yet thoroughly, and shape into burgers. Heat grill to medium-high and grill the burgers until no longer pink in the center, about 6 minutes on each side.

Ingredients

2 cloves garlic, finely minced ◆ 1 Tb grated ginger ◆ 1/4 cup chopped fresh cilantro ◆ 1/4 cup chopped fresh mint ◆ 1/4 cup chopped fresh basil ◆ 2 Tb lemon juice ◆ 1 Tb soy sauce ◆ 1 tsp sesame oil ◆ 1 tsp liquid sweetener ◆ 1 1/4 pounds ground turkey ◆ 1/3 cup soy nuggets or TVP

Stuffed Veal Loin

Butterfly veal, starting at one long side and cutting horizontally to within 1 inch of opposite long side. Open veal as if it were a book. Place a large sheet of plastic wrap over the veal and pound to 1/2-inch thickness, forming a rectangle approximately 10x12 inches. Discard plastic and season veal with salt and pepper. Combine soy cream cheese, chives, and roasted garlic in a bowl and beat until smooth. Blanch the basil leaves in boiling water until just wilted, drain, and rinse with cold water. Brush tomato paste along the center of the veal, forming a strip 2 inches wide. Spoon soy cream cheese mixture on top of tomato paste in an even log. Arrange basil leaves in an overlapping layer on top. Fold one long side of veal over filling and roll tightly. Cover ends of veal roil with heavy-duty aluminum foil to enclose filling completely. Tie kitchen string around veal rolls every 1 1/2 inches to maintain neat log shape. Wrap string lengthwise around veal roil to secure foil at ends, weaving string alternately under and over crosswise ties. Cover and refrigerate until well chilled, at least 6 hours. Preheat oven to 375° F. Heat olive oil in a large heavy roasting pan over medium-high heat. Season veal with salt and pepper, place in the pan, and brown on all sides, turning frequently, about 10 minutes. Remove pan from heat and cool veal for 15 minutes. Drape bacon slices over veal, tucking the ends under the roast. Roast veal in oven until a meat thermometer inserted into the center of the meat (not the filling) reads 140° F, about 45 minutes. Transfer to work surface and let stand 15 minutes. To serve, remove bacon, string, and foil from veal roast. Cut roast crosswise into even slices.

Ingredients

1 center-cut veal rib roast (rack of veal) ◆ about 4 1/2 lbs. boned and trimmed of all fat and outer membrane ◆ salt and pepper ◆ 1 container soy cream cheese ◆ 2 Tb chives ◆ 1 oz roasted garlic ◆ 16 large fresh basil leaves ◆ 2 Tb tomato paste ◆ 1 Tb olive oil ◆ 8 slices bacon

Sunset Barbecued Chicken

If you are using a charcoal grill, ignite 60 briquets on the grate of a barbecue with a lid. When briquets are dotted with gray ash (15-20 minutes after lighting), push them into two mounds on opposite sides of the grate. Set a drip pan on the grate between the mounds of charcoal. If you are using a gas grill, turn all burners to high and close the lid for 10 minutes. Adjust the burners for indirect cooking (heat on opposite sides of the grill rather than down the center). Keep heat on high. If you are using an oven broiler, heat oven (not broiler) to 450° F/200° C. Rinse chicken and pat dry. Set chicken on grill, not directly over heat. Cover the grill and open the vents. (Or place chicken in a foil-lined pan and roast) for 20 minutes. While the chicken is pre-cooking, whisk the remaining ingredients together in a small bowl. (If you are using an oven broiler, remove chicken from oven and pre-heat the broiler.) Brush half this mixture on top of the chicken. Return chicken to heat for 5 minutes. Turn chicken and baste underside with the remaining sauce. Cook until meat is no longer pink at the bone in the thickest part (about 5 minutes). The mustard coating should not be burnt.

Ingredients

2-3 lbs chicken pieces skin on ◆ 1 tsp liquid sweetener ◆ 2 Tb Dijon-style mustard ◆ 1 Tb Worcestershire sauce ◆ 1 tsp grated fresh ginger ◆ 1 clove garlic pressed ◆ salt and pepper to taste

Tofu, Scrambled

Squeeze water out of the tofu. Crumble tofu and mix with herbs and spices - add enough to make the tofu yellow and fragrant. Allow to sit for twenty minutes in the fridge.Heat a small pan with the zero-calorie butter spray. Add tofu mixture and a little water. Allow water to evaporate and the mixture to intensify in flavor, about 5-10 minutes, depending on how much water you put in. Remove from heat. Measure 4 ounces and serve.

Ingredients

1/4 pound extra-firm organic tofu ◆ zero-calorie butter spray ◆ curry powder ◆ thyme ◆ marjoram ◆ cumin ◆ salt ◆ black pepper ◆ ground red pepper ◆ garlic powder ◆ turmeric

Tofu, Stir Fried

Put entire package in freezer overnight. Thaw out one day in refrigerator. Remove tofu from package, and squeeze out all the water. Cut tofu into 1 inch cubes. Heat skillet at medium heat for 2-3 minutes. Spray zero-calorie butter spray in skillet. Add tofu. Stir occasionally to brown evenly for several minutes. Add seasoned salt toward end, so it doesn't burn. Weigh 4 oz. and serve. Refrigerate leftovers. Freezing tofu before cooking makes it nice and chewy!

Ingredients

1 package firm, or extra firm, tofu in water ◆ zero-calorie butter spray, abstinent seasoned salt

Tuna, Italian Pâté

Stir all ingredients together.

Ingredients

1/2 cup tuna ◆ allowable portion of unsalted butter, softened ◆ 3 teaspoons lemon juice ◆ salt and pepper

Turkey Bolognese

Heat oil in a sauté pan and fry garlic until it just turns golden. Add the ground turkey, sausage, and onion powder. Brown the meat, breaking it up as much as possible. Reduce heat and add vinegar, tomato paste, salt and pepper, and parsley. Simmer, stirring occasionally, for about 20 minutes. Stir in soy parmesan just before serving.

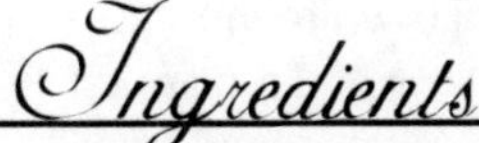

1 Tb olive oil ◆ 3 cloves garlic, minced ◆ 1 lb ground turkey ◆ 1 lb smoked sausage, sliced ◆ 1 Tb onion powder ◆ 3 Tb balsamic vinegar ◆ 2 Tb tomato paste ◆ 1 oz soy parmesan ◆ Salt and pepper ◆ 1 cup chopped parsley

Veal Scallopini Charleston

Combine lemon juice, Worcestershire sauce, mustard, vinegar, and parsley with 2 Tb of the oil and set aside. Heat remaining 1 Tb of the oil in a large sauté pan until it just starts to smoke. Coat the veal scallops with soy flour and season lightly with salt and pepper. Sauté quickly, allowing light brown color to form on veal. Transfer the veal onto a serving dish. Add the lemon juice mixture to the pan; when it is hot, add prosciutto and crabmeat. Toss until all is heated through, then pour over veal. If the veal has cooled in the interim, return veal to pot rather than pouring sauce over veal.

Ingredients

8 2-oz veal scallopini, pounded flat ◆ soy flour or soy bran ◆ salt and pepper ◆ 1 cup crabmeat ◆ 2 oz prosciutto crudo cut into thin strips ◆ 1 Tb lemon juice ◆ 1 tsp Worcestershire sauce ◆ 1 tsp mustard ◆ 1 Tb white vinegar ◆ 1 Tb chopped parsley ◆ 1 Tb olive oil

Warm and Hearty Breakfast

Sprinkle apple with cinnamon and bake in microwave for 3-5 minutes. Soak soy granules in water to soften them. (Pour just enough water to cover them, and depending on how quickly the water is absorbed, you may add a little more water.) Cut cheese into tiny chunks. Scramble egg and cheese into soy granules. Add apple into the mixture, and cook in microwave for another 3 minutes, or until the egg is no longer runny.

Ingredients

1 ounce texturized soy protein ◆ 1 egg ◆ 1/2 ounce Gjetost cheese ◆ 1 chopped apple ◆ cinnamon and sweetener

Winter Squash Souffle

Puree cooked squash, and season as usual with salt and pepper, adding a pinch of nutmeg and cinnamon. Beat eggs in a bowl until thoroughly mixed. Spray shallow glass or foil casserole dish with zero-calorie butter spray Pour beaten eggs into baking dish. Fold in squash until mixed with eggs. Bake at 350 degrees for 25 minutes, or until nicely puffed and browned.

Ingredients

2 eggs ◆ 1/2 cup winter squash ◆ zero-calorie butter spray ◆ salt ◆ pepper ◆ cinnamon ◆ nutmeg

3 raws Dip

Process all ingredients in food processor. Microwave to melt cheese and meld flavors (couple minutes on high usually). Dip your 3 raws to your heart's content.

Ingredients

3 oz canned soybeans ◆ 1 oz soycheese (any kind, I like pepperjack/cheddar combo) ◆ onion powder ◆ garlic powder ◆ celery seed powder ◆ hot pepper flakes ◆ 4oz rotel tomatoes (these are canned tomatoes w/green chili peppers) ◆ include some of the juice when you measure to make the dip spread smoother ◆ 1/2 t salt (or to taste) ◆ 4 oz canned mushrooms

A Dip for Steamed Broccoli

Mix some yogurt with French's salad mustard and balsamic vinegar.

Ingredients

yogurt ◆ French's salad mustard ◆ balsamic vinegar.

ABS Ice Cream

Mix in bowl then add to ice cream maker. Mix for 20 minutes depends on brand of machine.

Ingredients

4 oz. Plain Yogurt ◆ 6 oz. Milk ◆ 5 Soy Nuts prefer salted ◆ 1 tablespoon Instant Coffee ◆ 1 tablespoon Maple no alcohol extract ◆ 5 packets Sweet & Low ◆ 5 packets Equal

Protein - Dairy - Soy

3 raws Dip

Process all ingredients in food processor. Microwave to melt cheese and meld flavors (couple minutes on high usually). Dip your 3 raws to your heart's content. Measure as vegetable and protein.

Ingredients

3 oz canned soybeans ◆ 1 oz soycheese (any kind, I like pepperjack/cheddar combo) ◆ onion powder ◆ garlic powder ◆ celery seed powder ◆ hot pepper flakes ◆ 4oz rotel tomatoes (these are canned tomatoes w/green chili peppers) ◆ include some of the juice when you measure to make the dip spread smoother ◆ 1/2 t salt (or to taste) ◆ 4 oz canned mushrooms

A Dip for Steamed Broccoli

Mix some yogurt with French's salad mustard and balsamic vinegar.

Ingredients

yogurt ◆ French's salad mustard ◆ balsamic vinegar

ABS Ice Cream

Mix in bowl then add to ice cream maker. Mix for 20 minutes depends on brand of machine.

Ingredients

4 oz. Plain Yogurt ◆ 6 oz. Milk ◆ 5 Soy Nuts prefer salted ◆ 1 tablespoon Instant Coffee ◆ 1 tablespoon Maple no alcohol extract ◆ 5 packets Sweet & Low ◆ 5 packets Equal

Abstinent Custard

Beat ingredients together in a bowl. Place custard cups in a baking pan and fill. Pour boiling water around custard cups. Bake at 350° for one hour; allow to cool before serving.

Ingredients

8 oz milk ◆ 1 egg ◆ 1 tsp lemon flavoring ◆ 4 pkg splenda ◆ 1 tsp lemon peel ◆ variation: 1 tsp cinnamon

Abstinent Italian Cheesecake

Preheat oven to 350 degrees. With a food processor, mix soy flour, 8 pkg Splenda and cinnamon together. Add vanilla and cream soda. The mixture will turn into the consistency of play dough. Divide mixture by 8, and with your hands, form into balls and then flatten into a disc. Thoroughly coat a mini 8 loaf pan with non-stick spray. Place the disc in the center of one of the loaf molds and line and shape with your fingers into a crust. In the food processor, combine yogurt (labne), ricotta cheese, egg, lemon peel, remaining Splenda and lemon flavor. Mix well. Divide by 8, and add ricotta mixture on top of crust. In a separate dish, mix an additional 2 tsp cinnamon to 4 pkgs Splenda. Sprinkle mixture on top of cheese cakes (You probably won't use all of it). Bake at 350 degrees for one hour. Let cool and then remove from the bowl. Put in the refrigerator and serve cold. This is freezable, and can be defrosted in the microwave.

Ingredients

32 oz strained yogurt or labne ◆ 8 oz ricotta cheese ◆ 4 oz egg ◆ 2 TB + 2 tsp lemon flavor ◆ 2 TB + 2 tsp lemon peel ◆ 32 + 8 + 4 pkgs Splenda ◆ 4 oz soy flour ◆ 2 TB + 2 tsp vanilla ◆ 1/4 c + 1 TB cinnamon ◆ 1/2 c diet cream soda

Abstinent Italian Pepper Biscuits

Preheat the oven to 400 degrees. In a food processor, mix flour, spices and salt. As the food processor is running, slowly add water until the mixture becomes dough and begins to form a ball. Divide the dough into two pieces and roll each into a ball. Spray your hands, the dough, and a wooden chopping block with olive oil non-stick cooking spray. Form a rope with your hands with one of the balls, and then cut the rope lengthwise into quarters. Each quarter is a biscuit -- form a circle and join together at the center with your thumb. Make 8 biscuits. Place on a tray, cover with aluminum foil and spray top and bottom with non-stick cooking spray. Bake at 400 degrees for 15-20 minutes, until they turn brown or to taste. The longer you keep them in, the browner and more crunchy they get.

Ingredients

2 oz soy flour ◆ 2 TB + 2 tsp warm water (1.3 oz) ◆ Olive oil non-stick cooking spray ◆ 1/4 tsp salt ◆ 1/2 tsp coarsely ground black pepper ◆ 1/4 tsp fennel seeds ◆ 1/4 tsp onion powder

Apple--Yogurt--Soynutbutter Breakfast

Mix together in bowl.

Ingredients

8 oz. apple (cut up) ◆ 6 oz. yogurt ◆ 1 oz. soynut butter ◆ 1 oz. crushed soynuts

Abstinent Scones

Mix the soy flour, buttermilk, lemon peel, vanilla, and 4 pkgs of Splenda together. Spray a small ziploc container with non-stick cooking spray, and spoon in the mix. Microwave for 5 minutes. Turn out the scone onto a plate. For the topping, mix 4 pkgs of Splenda, lemon flavoring and yogurt together. Spread on the top of the scone. Note: As a variation, add 2 oz of blueberries to the scone and have 6 oz of fruit as a compliment.

Ingredients

2oz soy flour ◆ 4oz buttermilk ◆ 1 tsp lemon peel ◆ 1 tsp vanilla ◆ 4 + 4 pkg Splenda ◆ 1 tsp lemon flavoring ◆ 2 oz labne or strained yogurt ◆ Variation: 2 oz blueberries; Non-Stick Cooking spray

BAKED APPLE AND RICOTTA

Just bake or microwave a large apple (i.e. Rome) until it's done (i.e. soft), add vanilla extract and sweetener if desired, then top the whole thing with a measured dollop of ricotta cheese, with a bit more extract and sweetener. The contrast between the hot apple and the cold ricotta is very nice - or you can micro the whole thing for a minute more after you add the ricotta.

Ingredients

Large apple ◆ vanilla extract ◆ sweetener ◆ ricotta cheese

Breakfast

Place milk, strawberries, vanilla flavor and 1 package sweetener in blender and blend well for a delicious shake. Place apple slices on a microwaveable plate or bowl and sprinkle Gjetost cheese on top, drizzle butterscotch flavor on top, cover and microwave until cheese melts and starts to brown. Take out and immediately top with Labne/strained yogurt and sprinkle with 1 package of sweetener.

Ingredients

8 oz. cold milk ◆ 1/2 oz. Gjetost cheese cut in small pieces ◆ 2 oz. Labne or strained yogurt ◆ 4 oz. frozen strawberries ◆ 4 oz. cooked apple slices ◆ Frontier butterscotch and vanilla flavor, ◆ 1 to 2 packets sweetener

Breakfast "muffins"

Blend ingredients. You can, also, use a little seltzer water, diet soda, ginger ale, etc. added to the batter. This 'fluffs' the finished product a bit and loosens the batter when you are trying to stir it all together. Bake these in a small loaf pan, coated with any abstinent no stick spray at 350-375 degrees for 35 to 40 minutes.

Ingredients

1 egg ◆ 1 oz. Soy Flour ◆ 1 oz. Ricotta ◆ 2 oz. your favorite fruit| ◆ Stevia for sweetener ◆ S. & A. free extracts

Breakfast Muffin

Mix all ingredients together to make batter. Bake in large muffin tins for approx. 30 minutes at 350 degrees

Ingredients

1 Egg ◆ 1 oz. Soy Flour ◆ 1 oz. Soy Nut Butter ◆ Stevia for sweetening ◆ 2 oz. Fruit of choice ◆ Flavoring of choice

Candy Bar

Mix together really well. Freeze.

Ingredients

1 oz. soy nuts ◆ 1 oz. soy nut butter ◆ 2 oz. thick yogurt or labne ◆ sesame seeds ◆ butter or sesame oil ◆ 1/2 oz. gjetost cheese

Cannoli

Fill "wheat germ pancake" (see previous recipe) with a mixture of ricotta cheese, vanilla extract, and preferred sweetener to taste. Roll up, and close with toothpick.

Ingredients

Ricotta Cheese ◆ Vanilla Extract ◆ Sweetener to taste

Carrot Cinnamon Puree

Measure 1/2 c cooked carrots. Combine with 1/2 c soy milk (a 1/4 protein).. Mix ingredients in glass blender. Add sufficient boiling water to blend. Blender.

Ingredients

3 large raw carrots cut small ◆ 1/2 cup soy milk ◆ salt ◆ ginger ◆ cinnamon ◆ pepper and sweetener ◆ boiling water

Cauliflower Au Gratin

Take 1 head fresh cauliflower, clean it by taking the leaves off and coring part of the hard center part out. Cook the cauliflower head in the microwave on Power 8 or High for 10 minutes, covered. Or Cook the cauliflower on the stove in a covered pot with a small amount of water to steam, about 25 minutes, until the cauliflower is soft. Remove the cauliflower from the pot. Weigh and measure 16 oz or 2 cups, if you are using for a 2 cup vegetable. Or weigh and measure 8 oz. or 1 cup if you are using it for a 1 cup vegetable. (What is left over can be put up in a container in the fridge for another easy pre-cooked, to be reheated meal vegetable.) Measure 1 tablespoons. olive oil. (Or 1 1/2 teaspoon olive oil if using for a 1 cup lunch vegetable) Measure 2 oz. grated parmesan cheese. (Or 1 oz. grated cheese if using for 1/2 lunch protein). Place the measured oil and the measured cheese on the measured cauliflower.

Ingredients

Cauliflower

Cheesecake recipe

Place the egg and cheese in blender with sweet and low (4) and extract. Spray glass dish with oil, grind up about 1/4 cup of TVP and tap it around the bottom and sides of the dish. Put the cheese mixture in the dish. Bake for about 20 minutes (until a toothpick comes out clean) at 350 degrees, leave in oven for 20 minutes with it turned off.

Ingredients

32 oz ricotta cheese ◆ 2 eggs ◆ soy granules or TVP ◆ oil spray ◆ flavor extract with no alcohol(lemon or almond is good) ◆ 4 sweet and low

Cheryl's Wheat Germ Journeycakes

Beat egg(s) in a bowl and add wheat germ and spices. Melt butter in a non-stick pan. Pour batter in to form 2 patties. (If 2 eggs are used, batter will be thin and the result will be something like a tortilla; if one egg is used with 4 Tb wheat germ, the patties will have the thickness of bread. Pan-fry until done and pour the remaining butter over the top. Good hot or cold. Variation: if you cook these in the microwave, they come out with a sponge-cake texture.

Ingredients

1 egg (or 2) ◆ 1-4 Tb wheat germ, spices of your choice ◆ 1 Tb butter/margarine/oil

Chili

Saute ground beef, drain black soy beans mix together. Add all spices, along with 2 oz tomato sauce. Simmer on low heat for about 15 mins.

Ingredients

4 oz black soy bean and ground beef ◆ 2 oz tomato sauce ◆ 1 tbs. chili powder ◆ onion flakes ◆ 2 equal ◆ 1 tbs. red pepper

COCONUT CUSTARD

Combine ingredients and put in loaf pan or ramekin. Bake 450 for 15 minutes; reduce oven to 325 and cook for 35 minutes or until knife comes out clean. Cool in refrigerator and add fruit on top for Breakfast. or have for dinner with a salad.

Ingredients

1 egg ◆ 8 oz milk ◆ mix with sweetener ◆ vanilla ◆ coconut extract,(Alcohol Free Extracts! I like Frontier) ◆ salt (pinch to pull out sweet)

Coconut Custard

Put in loaf pan or ramekin. Bake 450 for 15 minutes. Reduce oven to 325 and cook for 35 minutes or until knife comes out clean. Cool in Fridge and add fruit on top for breakfast or have for dinner with a salad.

Ingredients

1 egg ◆ 8 oz milk mix with sweetener ◆ vanilla ◆ coconut extract, (Alcohol Free Extracts! I like Frontier) ◆ salt (pinch to pull out sweet)

COCONUT CUSTARD

Combine ingredients and put in loaf pan or ramekin. Bake 450 for 15 minutes. Reduce oven to 325 and cook for 35 minutes or until knife comes out clean. Cool in fridge and add fruit on top for Breakfast or have for dinner with a salad.

Ingredients

1 egg ◆ 8 oz milk, mix with sweetener ◆ vanilla ◆ coconut extract,(Alcohol Free Extracts! I like Frontier) ◆ salt (pinch to pull out sweet).

Coffee Shakes

Blend a lot starting on low setting and working way up to the highest setting. Let it get really airy and frothy...you wont believe it's abstinent!!! It really seems like there is milk in it, but there isn't! I keep brewed de-cafe in the fridge in pourable Tupperware containers. When it's getting low I make a new pot and refrigerate that so I never run out of the brewed de-café. A shake is always available that way!

Ingredients

Black coffee, already brewed (the way I like it, but some people use instant crystals) ◆ Ice, 4 packets Sweet-n-Low (Optional. Do it to your own taste) ◆ Extracts

Cold Breakfast Cereal

Put entire mixture in large bowl and mix with 1 cup or more cold water.

Ingredients

3 oz soy granules ◆ 1 oz soy milk powder ◆ 1 cup strawberries or other fruit ◆ water

Crispy Tofu

Remove block of tofu from package. Discard soaking water. Wrap tofu in plastic wrap and put in freezer. Once frozen solid remove tofu from freezer and place on plate and put in the refrigerator to defrost. Once completely defrosted place tofu between 2 plates over sink and press together to remove liquid being careful not to press too hard to break the tofu. Next slice or cube tofu into desired size. Saute/fry tofu in oil. Brown on both sides until crispy.

Ingredients

1 package firm tofu ◆ oil for cooking ◆ spices are optional

Croutons

I use the large unflavored dry TVP chunks, break them in half with the tip of a knife and spray them with garlic flavored PAM cooking spray. After weighing them, I throw them on my salad and enjoy.

Ingredients

TVP

Dessert Recipe

I heat everything together except the yogurt, which I add to the mix after it's been nuked. If you nuke the gsetost cheese just until it starts to turn dark, it will be delicious. Refrigerate and when ready to eat, add the yogurt.

Ingredients

5 oz Gsetost cheese counts as 1 protein) ◆ 1 oz. Yogurt (counts as 1/2 a protein) ◆ 5 oz. soynut butter (counts as 1/2 a protein) ◆ 2 Tbs. Wheat Germ (counts as 8 oz. vegetable)(mixed with 1/4 cup or so of water) ◆ 1 oz. Pumpkin (which is weighed out as part of my 8 oz. salad) ◆ 1 teaspoon combined Butterscotch & Orange flavorings (no sugar, no alcohol) ◆ Pumpkin Spices

Deviled Eggs

Hard boil the eggs. When slightly cool, cut the hardboiled eggs in half Scoop out the yolk and put in a small bowl Mix the yolk with the olive oil, the mustard and the Tabasco. When thoroughly mixed, spoon the egg mixture back into the egg-white halves. Sprinkle with Paprika if you like.

Ingredients

2 hardboiled Eggs ◆ 2 tablespoons Olive Oil ◆ 1/4 - 1 teaspoon dry mustard or wet mustard to taste ◆ 1/2 - 1 teaspoon Tabasco sauce (what makes them a 'deviled' egg) (optional)

Discrete Protein

"This recipe works if you want to weigh and measure discretely with little effort (easy prep also). Bring with you mixed in a quiet container.Order your huge salad, and weigh or cup it. Order your favorite sugar-free salad dressing. Order sugar-free marinara or tomato sauce if the restaurant has it, in a small side dish. Measure your salad (easy). Measure your dressing (easy). Pour your cheese-wheat germ mixture on top. DONE! Add tomato sauce if desired... DELICIOUS!" Variations (endless) (substitute soy nuts for 1 oz parmesan cheese) (add equal to sweeten it up a bit) (pre-mix your own salad dressing or oil with wheat germ and cheese for even greater discretion and less effort at the table).

Ingredients

2 oz. Parmesan Cheese ◆ 1/8 cup Wheat Germ

Discrete Protein

I bring 1 oz of soy nuts/Bacos (Bacos are soy and are abstinent thru my sponsor but check with yours of course) with 1/4 cup Wheat Germ and 2 teaspoons Peanut Oil mixed) I bring 1 baggie of cut carrots/sun-dried tomatoes (again on tomatoes check with sponsor). I order a salad and cup it and then put the carrots on top OR I eat the carrots while waiting for the meal. I then order a protein, weigh out 3 oz and put my soy mix on it.

Ingredients

2 oz. Parmesan Cheese ◆ 1/8 cup Wheat Germ

Dreamsicle

I take 1 cup of low-fat yogurt, add in one peeled and quartered orange, some vanilla flavoring and artificial sweetener. I blend it up in my mini-food processor and freeze it overnight.

Ingredients

1 cup Low-Fat Yogurt ◆ 1 Orange ◆ Vanilla Flavoring ◆ Artifical Sweetener

Egg Delight

First mix ricotta cheese with flavoring of your choice and an equal in a bowl together. Then put strawberries, blueberries, or any other fruit you would like in a bowl and let it cook in microwave 1-2 minutes until soft. Spray fry pan with butter spray put egg in like an omelet. Then add cheese on top of egg and half the fruit. Fold over egg like an omelet and add remaining fruit on top after put in a dish.

Ingredients

1 Egg or 2 oz. Egg Beaters ◆ 2 oz. Ricotta Cheese ◆ 8 oz. Fruit

Egg Delight

First mix together ricotta cheese with flavoring of your choice and an Equal in a bowl. In a separate bowl, cook fruit in microwave for 1-2 minutes until fruit is soft. In another bowl, beat egg with fork, like for scrambled eggs. Spray fry pan with butter spray. Put egg in pan and let set like an omelet. Add ricotta cheese mixture and half the fruit on top of egg. Fold over egg like omelet. Put out onto a plate and add remain cheese and fruit on top.

Ingredients

1 egg or 2 ozs. egg beaters ◆ 2 ozs. ricotta cheese ◆ 8 ozs fruit ◆ 1 Equal

Eggplant Parmesan

Cut an eggplant up either in rounds or lengthwise use about 2 tablespoons olive oil. Rub into the eggplant use Kosher salt, salt the eggplant well. Put in a baking dish on 350 in the oven for 30 minutes. Then add about 1/2 a jar of Classico Four Cheeses Spagetti sauce. Let cook another 30 minutes.

Ingredients

Eggplant ◆ 2 tablespoons Olive oil ◆ Kosher salt ◆ 1/2 jar Classico Four Cheeses Spagetti Sauce

Farmer Cheese Omelet

Spray bottom of large fry pan and heat it. Pour eggs into the pan and let cook. Spread and smear farmer cheese all over evenly and let cook a bit more until it looks blended. Fold over the thing into an omelet so the outside is browned and crisp. Flip. Slice into appropriate serving. (4 oz). For breakfast, add warm berries or other fruit on top.

Ingredients

4 seriously whipped eggs ◆ 4 oz. Farmer Cheese, creamy kind (or large curd whole milk cottage cheese) ◆ non-stick spray ◆ Cinnamon if you like it (or extract if you want it sweet)

Favorite Breakfast

Put diet soda, equal and salt in a small desert dish and fold with a fork, then put the dish containing liquid on the scale; set the scale to zero. Add the soy nut butter and blend vigorously with a fork until the soy nut butter is liquid; add in the ricotta cheese and blend with a fork; sprinkle the soy nuts on top of the completed mixture.

Ingredients

2.5 oz. ricotta cheese ◆ 5 oz. soy nut butter ◆ .5 oz. soy nuts ◆ 2 tbs diet soda ◆ 3 packets equal ◆ dash salt

Filling Breakfast

Heat apples - set aside. Mix yogurt with flavoring and sweeter - set aside. Take 1 oz. of soy flour and mix together cinnamon, and sweetener (optional), vanilla extract (or any flavor you like), and approximately 1/4 cup hot water. The consistency should be sticky like "cake dough". Add more water if necessary. Spray a round glass dish with "Pam" spray, and pour the dough in the pan. Microwave it for about 3 1/2 to 4 minutes. Take it out and put it on a plate. Top with 1/2 oz. shredded gjotost cheese, 8 oz. apples and 4 oz. yogurt. Microwave

Ingredients

4 oz. yogurt ◆ 1/2 oz. gjotost cheese ◆ 1 oz. soy flour ◆ 8 oz. apples (cooked) ◆ sweetener ◆ vanilla extract ◆ 1/4 cup hot water

French Onion Dip

Puree the cottage cheese into a paste, mixed it with the soup mix and sweetener. Let it sit in the fridge to absorb the flavors over night. Serve with raw finger vegetables.

Ingredients

1/2 cup cottage cheese ◆ 1 tablespoon french onion soup mix ◆ 1 packet sweetener

Fried Tofu

Get extra firm tofu at health food store and cut in cubes. Microwave for a long time until hard and chewy.

Ingredients

Tofu

Frozen Ricotta

Weigh out ricotta. Mix in cinnamon, sweetener, flavored coffee grinds and wheat germ portion. Coffee grinds-using less than 1/8 teaspoon of flavored coffee, like Hazelnut, adds an awesome taste to yogurt, ricotta, milk etc. Grind beans finely If you like extracts put that in too. Put in freezer. You can make ahead of time too. Don't have to eat right away.

Ingredients

3 oz Ricotta Cheese ◆ 1 oz Soy Nut Butter ◆ 1/8 cup Wheat Germ or 1/4 cup Wheat Germ - depending if you want to use 1/2 cup of a cooked vegetable (which I do if I am having it a dinner- whereby I put the cooked vegetable on top of my salad) ◆ Flavored Coffee Grinds

GINGERBREAD LOAF

Mix together all ingredients. Bake at 350 for 1/2 hour or so.

Ingredients

1 egg ◆ 1 oz wheat germ ◆ 2 oz. Soy flour or soya powder ◆ vanilla ◆ diet or club soda ◆ 1 tbs. fresh ginger ◆ cinnamon ◆ nutmeg ◆ sweetener ◆ flavoring

gjetost

Slice cheese into 1/4 inch slices and fry in a non stick pan. Mush it up with a spatula or it will burn. Form into a pancake shape. Drain on paper towels. Refrigerate until hard. Crumble up and use in grey sheet ice cream (tastes like caramel chips!) or use it with soy nuts as a trail mix.

Ingredients

gjetost

Gjetost Cheese Wheat Germ Cookie

Cut up the cheese in a small Tupperware container and add the peanut oil. Microwave for about 40 seconds (watch it so that it will not burn), then add the wheat germ and other ingredients. Mix well with the diet soda, just enough to make it moist but not too watery. Microwave for another 1 to 2 minutes. Freeze for about 15 minutes.

Ingredients

2 oz. cheese ◆ 1 oz. wheat germ ◆ 1 tablespoon peanut oil ◆ cinnamon ◆ sweetener ◆ diet soda for consistency

Greysheet Pizza

Measure out soy flour and put in a mini food processor or mixer with a dough hook. Add scant water just to let the dough gather into a ball. Press the dough into a small, flat bottomed Pyrex dish that has been sprayed with Pam and cook for approximately 2 minutes..Spread 1 oz. ricotta cheese on top of cooked dough. Spoon 2oz. (removed from the cooked veggie allowance) or stewed tomatoes, mashed, or tomato sauce on top of ricotta. Sprinkle grated Parmesan cheese on top of that...Add salt, pepper and garlic salt to taste over top. Microwave for 2-3minutes...till the cheese gets a little bubbly. Enjoy! This counts for 4oz. protein serving and 1/4 of cooked veggie serving. So room left for more cooked veggie and salad as well.

Ingredients

2oz Soy flour ◆ 1 oz. Ricotta cheese ◆ Water ◆ 1/2 oz. grated Parmesan cheese ◆ Salt ◆ Pepper ◆ Garlic salt to taste

GS Ice cream delicious

Mix ingredients in bowl. Keep bowl in freezer for at least 20 minutes.

Ingredients

240 gr (8 oz) of milk ◆ 2 tablespoons liquid sweetener ◆ 1 to 2 tablespoons flavoring (sugar-free and alcohol free)

Homemade Ice Cream

Mix ingredients in a blender until frothy and pour into a chilled (for 48 hours) ice cream bowl of an icecream maker. In 20 minutes, you should have ice cream. Scoop out the ice cream and serve with your remaining protein (1oz if you get 4 and more if you qualify). I measure out 1oz of soy nuts or 1/2 oz soynut butter and 1/2 oz soy nuts and sprinkle on top of my ice cream served with my remaining 4oz of fruit (an apple goes really well with the soynut butter).

Ingredients

12 oz milk (skim milk is best) ◆ 4oz peaches ◆ 5-7 equals or any other sweetener you prefer
◆ 1tsp of you favorite flavoring (to add interest)

Homemade Yogurt

Take 1 quart milk cold. Heat in the microwave 2 minutes 45 seconds. (You can test this on your microwave or stovetop). Or Heat on Stove top until the marker on the attached plastic tablespoon-with-thermometer that comes with the Yogurt Maker Set reads about 110 degrees. When the milk is heated to the right temperature, add 2 tablespoons readymade Plain yogurt with active yogurt cultures. Stir easily and swiftly with a whisk or spoon so the yogurt blends easily throughout the milk. Use a ladle or cup to pour the yogurt mixture into the (5) individual cups. Put the individual cups in the Yogurt Maker Base Frame to cook-ferment. Plug in the Yogurt Maker. Wait 7 hours. Viola fresh homemade yogurt. Put glass containers in fridge to cool and set.

Ingredients

1 quart cold milk ◆ 2 tablespoons Plain Yogurt

Ice cream

Put the cut up fruit in food processor, add the yogurt, sweetener to taste, and a cup or a bit more of crushed ice. Process for 10 seconds or until mixed. Put the whole thing into a bowl and put in the freezer for 15-20 minutes. Sprinkle top with hot Cajun chopped soynuts.

Ingredients

8 oz. fruit ◆ 1 oz. yogurt ◆ 1/2 oz. of Cajun spiced soy nuts ground up

Karen's Wheat Germ Muffin

Place 2 or 4 Tb wheat germ in Rubbermaid™ size 0 or comparably small container. Add about 2 Tb water, sweetener, and spices. Microwave uncovered for about 4 minutes. Wheat germ should puff up into a muffin shape. The time required to get this properly cooked will depend on the strength of your microwave: if it isn't done in 4 minutes, cook it longer. Spread the butter on afterwards.

Ingredients

2 or 4 Tb wheat germ ◆ 1 Tb butter ◆ allspice ◆ cinnamon ◆ sweetener

Looks like Cheesecake Dessert

Take wheat germ, melted butter and small amount extract, mix and flatten on bottom of bowl. Add soy nut butter and mix into wheat germ and flatten. Add yogurt mixed with some extract to top and sprinkle with nuts. Should be in kind of layers. Chill.

Ingredients

5 oz strained plain yogurt ◆ 1 oz soy nut butter ◆ 5 oz soy nuts ◆ 1 oz wheat germ ◆ 1T Butter ◆ vanilla extract

Mock "Thai peanut sauce"

Combine all ingredients in blender or food processor. Mix until smooth. Makes one cup prepared.

Ingredients

1/2 cup soynut butter ◆ 1/3 cup firm silken tofu (drain or squeeze out liquid) ◆ legal equivalent of 3T sugar (substitute) ◆ 2 T fresh lime juice ◆ 2 T tamari sauce ◆ 1/2 to 3/4 tsp crushed red pepper, to taste ◆ 2 garlic cloves.

Mock French Toast

Mix ingredients together with a hand beater until frothy. Pour into a small skillet sprayed with Pam and cover. Cook over low heat until set. Remove and sprinkle with sweetener and cinnamon to taste.

Ingredients

1 large egg ◆ 1/4 cup ricotta cheese ◆ 1 teaspoon vanilla ◆ cinnamon and nutmeg to taste

Mock French Toast

Mix with a hand beater until frothy. Pour into a small skillet sprayed with Pam and cover. Cook over low heat until set. Remove and sprinkle with sweetener and cinnamon to taste.

Ingredients

1 large egg ◆ 1/4 cup ricotta cheese ◆ 1 teaspoon vanilla ◆ cinnamon and nutmeg to taste

Mock Frozen Soy Brittle

Mix together really well and freeze. Freeze

Ingredients

1 oz. soy nuts ◆ 1 oz. soy nut butter ◆ 2 oz. thick yogurt or labne ◆ sesame seeds ◆ butter or sesame oil ◆ 1/2 oz. gjetost cheese

Muesli

Mix and serve.

Ingredients

1/2 cup yogurt ◆ 2 ounces soy nuts ◆ 1/8 cup wheat germ ◆ 1 tablespoon peanut, walnut, or hazelnut oil (optional from fat measurement) or abstinent extract, to taste (vanilla, chocolate, almond)

Muffins

Mix together and put in muffin tin sprayed with Pam. Bake for about 30 minutes

Ingredients

2 oz soy flour ◆ 1 egg ◆ 4 oz carrots ◆ cinnamon ◆ nutmeg ◆ stivia or equal ◆ alcohol free extract (vanilla/almond your preference) ◆ diet soda as liquid

Mushrooms, Onions, and "Barley"

Cover TVP with boiling water until all liquid is absorbed. Cook onions in Pam. Measure out. Cook mushrooms and measure. Add to TVP with rest of ingredients.

Ingredients

1 oz. TVP ◆ ¼ cup sautéed onions ◆ 1/2 cup sautéed mushrooms ◆ 1 tbs. Butter ◆ salt

Mushrooms, Onions, and Soy

Cover texturized soy protein with boiling water until all liquid is absorbed. Spray skillet with zero-calorie butter spray. Cook onions and mushrooms in skillet, until onions are clear. Measure 1/2 cup. Add vegetables and measured portion of butter with texturized soy protein and mix. Warms your tummy!

Ingredients

1 ounce texturized soy protein ◆ 1/4 cup sautéed mushrooms ◆ 1/4 cup sautéed onions ◆ butter zero-calorie cooking spray ◆ salt

Pasta, soy

Reserve up to 2 oz of soy for flouring of board. Mix egg and few drops of water well and salt, add 4 oz soy beat till a stiff ball forms. You may need to add drops of water to make it all pick up into the ball. You will use your hands in this. When it all comes together yet is wet enough to be workable set aside and cover to keep wet. Cut off small piece and dust it with the remaining flour, and the rolling pin and your knife, hands. Be very careful with where you put and how you use the reserve, as it all has to be used up. This will come with practice. Roll out strip to thinness desired. Lay on a next plate, tray or something TO DRY. Repeat till all is done. Any remaining, add a bit of water and use up. Let dry till very dry. Depending on climate could take half a day or so. Divide into 2 equal parts and zip lock and freeze or save or use. Cooking. In deep boiling, salted water boil for short period of time, about 4 minutes, test. Serve with tom sauce. Can also be cut in pasta machine, following regular method, but keep it sort of thick. It requires too much dusting to become very thin and it is not very pliable dough.

Ingredients

6 oz soy ◆ salt ◆ 1 egg ◆ few drops of water as needed only.

Pineapple Yogurt Ice Cream

Blend ingredients in blender, and work up in ice cream maker; add crunchy TVP when ice cream is nearly done. Blender, ice cream maker. Freeze.

Ingredients

6 oz. yogurt ◆ 8 oz. chunk pineapple ◆ 1 Equal ◆ vanilla flavoring ◆ TVP

Quiche

Mix together well. Spray the bottom of a plastic dish generously. Nuke for a long time till all done and a but browned. Measure out your 4 oz. after it is cooked.

Ingredients

Eggs whipped ◆ Ground pork or meat already cooked ◆ Soy cheese grated or cubed

Quickie breakfasts 1

Microwave about 30 to 40 seconds. Eat with fruit.

Ingredients

1 1/2 oz. ghetost ◆ cut up small ◆ 1 oz. soy nuts ◆ flavoring/sweetener to taste

Quickie breakfasts 2

Blend in blender.

Ingredients

1/2 cup yogurt or 2 oz ricotta ◆ 1 cup milk ◆ morning fruit or flavoring ◆ sweetener optional

Quickie breakfasts 3

Microwave on high for 1 minute. Add fruit if desired.

Ingredients

2 oz. TVP ◆ 1 cup milk ◆ optional sweetener or flavorings

Rich Blue Cheese Dressing

Take sour cream, whole milk and blue cheese and mix together.

Ingredients

3 tbs sour cream ◆ 1/4 c whole milk ◆ 1.375 oz. Blue Cheese

Ricotta & Yogurt Dip/Dressing

Combine equal amounts (or nearly equal, so it adds up to total protein serving) of ricotta cheese and yogurt. Add and mix in your favorite herbs and spices.

Ingredients

Ricotta cheese ◆ yogurt ◆ favorite herbs and spices ◆ tomato paste or sauce for extra zing

Ricotta Combo

Mix as much of each ingredient as you want until you hit the 4 oz.(or your protein allotment) on the scale. It comes out as a nice, firm mixture that I stuff inside a half cantaloupe or 1/4 honeydew. Add sweetener to each ricotta combo, if you like.

Ingredients

Ricotta, white soft farmer cheese (the 4 oz. kind not the hard one that's a 2 oz. cheese) ◆ cottage cheese ◆ soy ream cheese ◆ grated hard ricotta salata (it's a four ounce protein for me but check with your sponsor before using in the mixture).

Roasted Soynuts

Soak your beans covered in water for at least 12 hours or over n night. Drain. Spread them out on a cookie sheet in a single row, or as single as possible. Spray with a little non-stick or use a spray of oil. I added same salt and garlic powder. Cook at 325 for 1-3 hours stirring occasionally. They should get brown and crunchy. Or if you like them a little softer stop sooner. You can't taste for doneness. Squeeze a nut and see how it goes.

Ingredients

Soy Nuts

Sallie's Standard Soya Bake

Combine dry ingredients in a large bowl and mix thoroughly, using your hands as little as possible. Add water a few Tb at a time until mixture forms a dryish ball in the center of the bowl. (The texture should be rather like that of pie dough. You may also use a food processor to do this.) Place dough on a foil-lined tin and press into a circle or rectangle about 1 1/2 inches thick. Bake at 180°C for 30-40 minutes, until well done.

Ingredients

2 oz soy flour ◆ 2 oz soy bran ◆ 1/4 cup wheat germ ◆ salt ◆ pepper ◆ thyme ◆ paprika ◆ 1 tsp liquid sweetener

Smoked Gouda and Onion Wheat Germ Quiche

Pre-heat oven to 375. Melt the butter in a small skillet. Set aside. Bake the empty wheat germ pie shell for 5 minutes. Remove from the oven and place it on a cookie sheet. You can use aluminum tins purchased at the grocery store for the quiche tins. Place the cheese in the bottom of the warm shell. In a mixing bowl, lightly beat the egg. Whisk in the milk, parsley, onion flakes, and seasonings. Pour into the shell. Bake for 20-30 minutes, or until the pie is firm. Serve warm or chilled.

Ingredients

1 tablespoon Butter ◆ 1/2 oz. dried Onion flakes ◆ 1/2 tsp dried Parsley flakes ◆ 2 tablespoons Wheat Germ (pressed and frozen in a tin or dish) ◆ 1/2 oz Smoked Gouda Cheese, grated (1/4 GS protein) ◆ 1 Egg (1/2 GS protein) ◆ 1/2 cup Milk (1/4 GS protein) ◆ Dash White Pepper ◆ 1/8 teaspoon Salt

Soy Brittle Bar

Mix together really well. Freeze.

Ingredients

1 oz. soy nuts ◆ 1 oz. soy nut butter ◆ 2 oz. thick yogurt or labne
Sesame seeds ◆ butter or sesame oil ◆ 1/2 oz. gjetost cheese

Soy Butter Variation

Mix ingredients together. Heat in microwave almost one minute, to this hot concoction add 1/2 cup thick creamy natural yogurt.

Ingredients

1/4 cup Wheat Germ ◆ 2 oz Soy butter ◆ 1 tablespoon Butter or margarine ◆ 1/4 cup Black coffee (cold is okay)
◆ 1/2 cup thick creamy natural Yogurt

Soy Loaf

You have to judge how much to use by how moist the batter becomes. I would practice a few times to get the right mix. The batter needs to be moist. Spice as you like it (garlic powder, cinnamon, vanilla or whatever flavor you fancy and/or sweetener depending on whether you want a sweet or spicy muffin). Spray a loaf pan or a muffin tin with Pam and pour in the batter and bake at 400; 15 minutes (muffins) – 25 minutes for a loaf. It should be brown and crispy on top remove carefully sometimes they stick.

Ingredients

2oz soy flour ◆ 1 egg ◆ 1 teaspoon baking soda (not powder) ◆ 4-6 oz vegetable (pumpkin, zucchini, virtually anything that is already cooked)

Soy Lunch On The Go

Mix all ingredients except for milk and soy nuts in a bowl with a little water or Diet Crème soda. Microwave to melt. Then mix in Soy Nuts. Milk can be mixed in also but I prefer to have 2 oz milk with coffee. Trust me this is incredible with a cup of coffee. This can be stored in the fridge or freezer. It travels well.

Ingredients

1 oz. Gjetost cheese cut into small pieces ◆ 1 oz. Soy Butter ◆ 1 oz. Wheat germ ◆ 1/2 tsp. unsweetened Cocoa powder or 1/2 tsp. chocolate flavor ◆ 1/2 tsp. butterscotch flavor ◆ 1 Tblsp Hazelnut Oil ◆ 1/2 oz. Soy nuts ◆ 2 oz. milk

Soy Muffins for Plane Travel

Mix to make it all wet, but not soupy. Microwave until firm.

Ingredients

3 oz soy ◆ 2 oz milk ◆ 1 oz wheat germ
◆ sweetener and extract to taste ◆ diet soda

Soy Nut Butter "Fudge"

Put all ingredients in a bowl. Heat for 20 secondss in the microwave. Stir it all up until semi-smooth. Put in freezer for minimum 30-40 minutes.

Ingredients

1 1/2 oz Soy Nut Butter ◆ 1 1/2 oz Ricotta Cheese ◆ 1/2 oz Gjetost Cheese ◆ 1 Tb. Peanut Oil ◆ 1 oz. Wheat Germ ◆ Equal, etc. to taste ◆ Bickford or Frontier Flavors of choice

Soy Nuts from Soybeans

MSoak soybeans in water overnight. Drain. Take a very small amount of oil and and flavoring. salt. onion powder ,garlic powder or plain and toss with beans. Roast at 350 for about 2 hours or more. Check and mix around. They need to be toasty and hard.

Ingredients

Soybeans

Soy Pancake

Combine 1 egg mixed with a certain amount of water, cinnamon, salt and sweet and low. (nothing else) Mix well. Add 2 oz soy flour. Mix/beat with fork/spoon till all the soy is well mixed. Mixture should be a perfect balance of flowing to pour and yet not runny. Start by adding small amounts of water and a thick batter and keep adding a few drops till you get a pouring consistency. Pour into hot Teflon fry pan sprayed with non-fat cooking spray. Lower heat just slightly and cover leaving a little crack open for steam. Cook quite a while on one side (don't go away, it willburn) . When you see lots of bubbles coming thru, carefully lift and see if it is dark and ready to turn. Turn, lower heat again and cover. Makes onelarge to die for I/House Pancake. Serve over fruit with other legal options if desired.

Ingredients

1 egg ◆ water ◆ cinnamon ◆ salt ◆ sweet and low ◆ 1 oz. Soy flour ◆ fruit

Soy Pancakes

Hot Teflon pan sprayed. Mix/beat with fork/spoon till all the soy is well mixed. Pan is now getting very hot. Mixture should be a perfect balance of flowing to pour and yet not runny. Start by adding small amounts of water and a thick batter and keep adding a few drops till you get a pouring consistency. Pour into hot fry pan and just slightly lower heat and cover with a crack open for steam. Cook quite a while on one side (don't go away, it will burn). When you see lots of bubbles coming thru, carefully lift and see if it is dark and ready to turn. Turn, lower heat again and cover. Makes one large to die for I/House Pancake. Serve over fruit with other legal options if desired.

Ingredients

1 egg ◆ a certain amount of water ◆ cinnamon ◆ salt and sweet and low. (nothing else) ◆ 2 oz soy flour.

Soy Pancakes

Beat the egg, add soy flour and all other ingredients except the seltzer. Add seltzer to make the consistency somewhat liquid. Heat frying pan with oil, butter or Pam, fry on one side, turn when browned on bottom. stovetop.

Ingredients

1 egg ◆ 1.5 oz. soy flour ◆ alcohol free vanilla ◆ dash of cinnamon ◆ lemon flavored seltzer ◆ sweetener to taste ◆ dash of lemon zest or orange zest ◆ 1 tablespoon sesame seeds

Soy Pancakes for Breakfast

Beat the egg, add soy flour and all other ingredients except the seltzer. Add seltzer to make the consistency somewhat liquid. (also works well with diet sprite, adjust sweetener). Heat frying pan with oil, butter or Pam, fry on one side, turn when brown on bottom.

Ingredients

1 Egg ◆ 1.5 oz. Soy flour ◆ alcohol free Vanilla ◆ dash of Cinnamon ◆ Lemon flavored seltzer ◆ Sweetener to taste ◆ dash of Lemon zest or Orange zest (from a spice jar, or grate your own) ◆ 1 tablespoon Sesame seeds (optional depending on line of sponsorship)

Soy Spaghetti

Take a glass baking dish. Either tear up or cut up some bacon (check ingredients on package - if it doesn't mention pork or bacon as an ingredient, ask your sponsor if you can count "pork" as ingredient #1. I don't think I've noticed any packs of bacon listing "bacon" or "pork" as an ingredient. There are completely sugarless bacons). Cook the bacon spread out on the dish in the oven so the pieces aren't touching, until it's released some of the grease but is still soft. Then mix in the soy product (the above product looks exactly like spaghetti, but there's probably other shapes/thicknesses available). Cook the mixture (I must've used a 350-degree oven) until the soy product is the way you like - some prefer it crisp, some don't. Doesn't take long (sorry to be so vague--abstinence forced me to learn to cook a little bit but not much). If you like it crispy, watch that the bacon doesn't burn. I would weigh 3-1/2 oz of the soy/bacon mixture onto a plate, saving 1/8 of my protein to be used as 1/4 oz of grated Parmesan cheese. Meanwhile I had heated up tomato sauce/spicy garlic sauce mixture in a saucepan and boiled up a bag of dark, dried mushrooms I also got in Chinatown (I used garlic vinegar in the boiling water). The tomato-mushroom preparation was measured for my cooked vegetable (1 cup or 8 oz), and I had the option of using up to a certain amount of additional sauce as 'condiment.' Add salt/pepper, if you like (I do). The grated Parmesan goes on top of the whole thing. This was so good I served it to "normal" eaters, who loved it! A dark green salad goes very well, and because of the greasiness of the bacon, you still have all your fat to use, as you like.

Ingredients

Stripped Tofu

Soy Stix

Mix one egg in a tall pitcher bowl. Add McCormick Montreal steak seasonings/salt, or your own spice mix. Add 2 oz soy flour. Beat well. Will form a dough ball and be dry/stiff. Take with hands and work into a ball. Lay on board and cut off small piece about 1/7th or 1/8. Roll as a child rolls play dough, like a snake on the board. Gets long and thin -- not too thin about 1/4" round. Cut into 3 pieces. Continue till all used up. Lay on round tray in Microwave oven. Cook at 3 minutes Power level 6 (mine Sharp Carrousel ?watts). Leave in Microwave a while for 1 or 2 minutes after finished to "set".

Ingredients

1 egg ◆ McCormick Montreal steak seasonings/salt(or your own spice mix) ◆ 2 oz soy flour

Soy Stix

Mix egg, seasons, spice and flower together in a tall pitcher bowl and beat well. Will form a dough ball and be dry/stiff. Take with hands and work into a ball. Lay on board and cut off small piece about 1/7th or 1/8. Roll as a child rolls play dough. Like a snake on the board. Gets long and thin -- not too thin about 1/4" round. Cut into 3 pieces. Continue till all used up. Lay on round tray in Microwave oven. Cook for 3 minutes at medium high. Leave in Microwave a while (1 or 2 minutes) after finished to "set". They can be used as is, dipped, or cut small into little things, Taste sort of like Dumplings. By the shape you make them, you can call them what you want. I even cut them up small and smother them in a tomato paste sauce and called it Pasta.

Ingredients

1 egg ◆ McCormick Montreal steak seasonings/salt(or your own spice mix) ◆ 2 oz soy flour

Soynut butter cookies

Combine all ingredients well. Bake at 350 for about 25-30 minutes.

Ingredients

.75 oz soy flour or powder ◆ 75 oz soynut butter ◆ 1 egg ◆ 1 oz yogurt ◆ 2 tb wheat germ ◆ 1 tb oil or butter ◆ cinnamon ◆ artificial sweetener to taste

Spinach, Egg, and Ricotta Bake

Mix all together. Spray a microwaveable bowl with Pam and bake for 6 minutes.

Ingredients

1 egg ◆ 1/4 cup ricotta ◆ 1/4 cup vadalia onions sauteed in olive oil ◆ 3/4 cup cooked spinach ◆ salt ◆ nutmeg ◆ ginger to taste

Strawberry Ice Cream

Refrigerate until very cold, then use ice cream machine as per directions.

Ingredients

16 oz whole milk ◆ 8 oz fresh strawberries ◆ 2 tsp. brown sweet and low ◆ 1 tbs alcohol-free vanilla

Strawberry Ice Cream

Mix in bowl then add to ice cream maker. Let ice creamer maker run for 20 minutes. Blender,freezer.

Ingredients

4oz plain yogurt, 6oz milk ◆ 5 soy nuts ◆ 1 tablespoon any flavor extract ◆ 1 tablespoon instant coffee if you like ◆ 5 sweet & low ◆ 5 Equal

Tanya's Soyabake

Combine ingredients with the seasonings of your choice and mold into a ball or loaf. Bake at 350°until done.

Ingredients

3 oz soy flour ◆ 1 oz soy nuts ◆ 2 or 4 Tb wheat germ ◆ 1 Tb peanut oil ◆ 1/2 cup water ◆ salt

Thick and Creamy Strained Yogurt w/Crushed Soy Nuts

Crush the soy nuts and set aside. Mix yogurt with sweetener and extract. Put in freezer for the few minutes so it gets amazingly perfectly chilled. Using paper towel or a cheesecloth strain the yogurt (just dump a whole container of yogurt into the cloth, which you have tightly fastened over a bowl that can catch the water/liquid that will be dripping/straining out of the yogurt. Cover this contraption with a piece of plastic wrap and stick it in the fridge and forget about it for a while. This takes a long time, so do it at least a day prior to it being your breakfast and you'll see how it gets thicker and thicker over time...I keep it in this bowl with the plastic wrap over it. Once you have it to your desired thickness measure it out as an 8 oz protein, yogurt.

Ingredients

6oz Strained Yogurt ◆ 1 oz Soy Nuts ◆ Non-alcohol Vanilla extract ◆ Non-alcohol Peanut Butter Extract ◆ 2 Sweet-n-Low

Vegetarian Smoky Cheesy Bacon & Eggs

Sprinkle veggies with salt and Dash and cook in olive oil until they start to brown. Weigh/measure cooked veggies into a bowl. Add wheat germ, bacon bits, cheese and egg and mix together. You can either nuke this to melt the cheese or place back in frying pan. This is also good minus the bacon bits or links and using 1oz. smoked cheddar instead of 1/2 oz. cheddar. Meat eaters could use real bacon or sausage.

Ingredients

1 egg ◆ 1/2 oz. Smoked Cheddar Cheese grated ◆ 1 oz. BADIA Imitation Bacon Bits (I have found this in the supermarket in the spice section) or 1 oz. cooked sliced Lightlife Lean Breakfast Links ◆ onions ◆ green cabbage ◆ baby carrots ◆ wheat germ ◆ olive oil ◆ Jane's Crazy Mixed Up Salt ◆ Mrs. Dash original flavor

Vanilla Cookies

Put all ingredients except soy powder into food processor. Add soy powder until mixture turns crumbly, then add a tiny bit of water until it turns into a ball of dough. Spray your hands with non-fat cooking spray and gather it together into a ball. You can chill this in fridge a little while to make it easier to work with, but its not absolutely necessary. Roll dough out between two pieces of wax paper or parchment paper. Roll until its very thin (1/8 inch) cut into shapes with cookie cutter. Place on cookie sheet sprayed with non stick cooking spray. Spray the cookies again lightly. Bake at 350 till lightly browned on edges. For Icing: Beat egg white till foamy, then add lots of splenda till mixture is stiff enough to put in pastry bag. Decorate cookies. You can thin this out, paint it on with a brush and then dust with splenda if you want that look.

Ingredients

Soy Powder (finer than soy flour- Fearns makes it) ◆ Egg ◆ Sweetener; SF, AF Vanilla extract (or any type you prefer) ◆ Baking powder (a dash)
Icing: Egg white ◆ Splenda (granulated kind for cooking and baking)

Warm Hearty Breakfast

Sprinkle apple with cinnamon and bake in microwave 3-5 minutes. Soak soy granules in water to soften them. (I pour just enough water to cover them and, depending on how quickly the water is absorbed, may add a little more water.) Cut cheese into mini-chunks. Mix in egg and cheese. Mix in apple mixture. Cook in microwave for another 3 minutes, or until egg is no longer runny.

Ingredients

1 oz soy granules ◆ 1 egg ◆ 1/2 oz cheese (I use Ghetost for this) ◆ 1 apple

Wheat Germ and Gjetost Cheese

Mix together. Store in freezer and either eat it alone or add it to fresh fruit or my gjetost baked apple. (1 apple baked with 1/2 oz. Gjetost, cinnamon and sweetener. Sometimes I add soy nuts to this dessert too.

Ingredients

1 oz. wheat germ ◆ 1/2 oz. Gjetost cheese ◆ 1 T butter.

Wheat Germ Cookie

Mix all together until you get a pretty thick paste. Microwave in the oven on a plate or in small cups, turning over from time to time. Watch carefully so they don't burn.

Ingredients

60 gm. wheat germ ◆ 40 gm. sesame seeds ◆ 60 gm. Tachini ◆ 1/2 cup water ◆ salt ◆ pepper ◆ tabasco

WHEAT GERM CUPCAKES

In a separate container (a Rubbermaid cup works well) mix the wheat germ with a few abundant shakes of ground cinnamon, ground ginger (less than cinnamon), and black pepper (less than ginger) and add the optional sesame seeds (some people use poppy seeds). If you don't like sweet or spicy food, try something else - like garlic salt and perhaps mild mustard seeds. Melt the butter in about 1/2 cup of hot tap water (1/4 cup if you're on 1/8 cup w.g.) and add liquid sweetener to taste. This is where you'd be able alternatively to use, e.g., garlic salt and mustard seeds. Stir the liquid into the dry mixture. Spray the baking tin with butter-flavored Pam or a similar product. Spoon the mixture into the baking receptacle. Bake it for a long time on low heat so it resembles what they used to give babies when they're teething! Since there's nothing in the ingredients that NEEDS cooking, the heat is just to make it firm enough to pick up.

Ingredients

1 oz wheat germ (my maintenance allowance - if you're on 1/8 cup wheat germ, halve the recipe) ◆ 1 tbsp butter or margarine ◆ 1/2 cup water ◆ 1 tbsp sesame seeds (check with sponsor) ◆ sweetener and/or spice if desired.

Wheat Germ Pancakes

Combine egg and wheat germ, and cook it like a pancake in a sprayed pan. You can also bake it in the bottom of a small loaf pan, in which case, it even takes on the shape of bread.

Ingredients

Eggs ◆ Wheat Germ

WHEATGERM MUFFIN

Add wheat germ and soy flour to egg. Mix with vanilla. Add diet soda or club soda to change texture. Bake at 350 for 1/2 hour or so.

Ingredients

1 egg ◆ 1 oz wheat germ ◆ 2 oz. Soy flour or soya powder ◆ vanilla ◆ diet or club soda.

Yogurt Mix

Take plain yogurt and mix in 1 serving of favorite fruit (sweetened).

Ingredients

1 cup (8 oz.) yogurt plain ◆ unsweetened ◆ 1 serving of fruit ◆ sweetener

Wisdom

DENMW
Don't Eat No Matter What

The Last Resort
This is the last resort of last resorts

The Last House on the Block
Greysheet is the last house on the block

G.O.D.
Good Orderly Direction
Gift of Desperation

Keep Your Eyes of Your Own Plate
I keep my eyes on my own plate.

It's not Mine

Abstinent & Grateful
I'm abstinent and grateful.

Nothing Tastes As Good As Abstinence Feels

Failing to Plan is Planning to Fail

Shopping and Chopping

Don't Give Up Before the Miracle

Let Me Cultivate an Attitude of Gratitude

Today I Must Live

Thy Will, Not Mine Be Done

The Only Way:
Surrender to 3 Weighed & Measured Meals a Day

Half Way Measures Avail Us Nothing

I Am Worth It

If You Feel God is Far Away, Guess Why Moved?

I Am Responsible

Hurt People Hurt Other People

The Great Thing in the World
Is not so much where we stand,
As in What Direction we are Moving

Success: If you've tried to do something
And failed, you're vastly better off than
If you'ld tried to do nothing and succeeded

It All Begins Today

Step Zero: Put Down the Food

With You, I'm Me

With you I feel that I can be
    Happy, Joyous and Free
I Open up my heart to you
    In simple honesty.
I share my inner thoughts
    Abandon all disguises
I bare my deepest feelings
    Shunning pretense or surprises
I stand before you as I am,
    My strengths and flaws revealed:
No attitudes are hidden,
    No motives are concealed.
With you I'm free to be myself,
    Voice my identity.
I draw from you an inner clam
    That says with you, I'm me.

We can Do What I Can't

This is a We Program
I Can't; He Can, and I Am Going to Let Him

As the Swan Swims on the Lake

With head high -
It appears that she has it made
But her feet are working like mad
To swim!
As in Greysheet - the people who seem
To have it made
Are working like mad
To keep their abstinence
One Day at a Time!

No Fight - No Victory

I Have Been Blessed

With enough pain–to allow me to feel to the fullest, the joy of living.

With enough problems–to help me grow to my fullest potential in this life.

With enough character defects–to keep me humble when experiencing the defects of others.

With enough turmoil–so that I can fully enjoy the quiet times of my life

With enough rejection–so that I can fully appreciate the unconditional love that I find in my new life.

With enough fear–to teach me the peacefulness of faith

I have been specially blessed with enough program to Realize that my happiness is MY responsibility and is achieved by MY improving on MY character defects.

H.A.L.T

Don't get too hungry, angry, lonely, or tired

We Realize

Others are frequently wrong and often sick.

--12 Steps

We are not primarily put on
this earth to see through
one another, but to see
one another through.

Serenity is Not
Freedom from the Storm,
But Peace Amid the Storm

Self Pity is An Alibi for Inaction
Anger is Danger

The Promises
We are going to know a new freedom
and a new happiness.
We will not regret the past
nor wish to shut the door on it.
We will comprehend the word
Serenity and we will know peace
No matter how far down the scale we
have gone, we will see how our experience
can benefit others.
That feeling of uselessness and self-pity will disappear.
We will lose interest in selfish things
and gain interest in our fellows.
Self-seeking will slip away.
Our whole attitude and outlook on
Life will change.
Fear of people and of economic insecurity
will leave us.
We will intuitively know how to handle
situations which used to baffle us.
We will suddenly realize that
God is doing for us what we could not
do for ourselves.

Just for Today
Just for Today I will try to live through this day only, and not tackle my whole life problem at once. I can do something for twelve hours that would appall me if I felt I had to keep it up for a lifetime.

Just for Today I will be happy. This assumes to be true what Abraham Lincoln said, that "Most folks are as happy as they make up their minds to be."

Just for Today I will adjust myself to
what is, and not try to adjust everything
to my own desires. I will take my "luck"
as it comes, and fit myself to it.

Just for Today I will try to strengthen
my mind. I will study. I will learn something
Useful. I will not be a mental loafer.
I will read something that requires effort,
thought and concentration.

Just for Today I will exercise my soul
in three ways: I will do somebody a good
turn, and not get found out; if anybody
knows of it, it will not count. I will do at
least two things I don't want to do–just for exercise.
I will not show anyone that my feelings are hurt:
they may be hurt, but today I will not show it.

Just for Today I will be agreeable.
I will look as well as I can, dress becomingly,
talk low, act courteously, criticize not one bit,
not find fault with anything and not try to improve
or regulate anybody except myself.

Just for Today I will have a program.
I may not follow it exactly, but I will have it.
I will save myself from two pests: hurry and
indecision.

Just for Today I will have a quiet half
hour all by myself, and relax. During this
half hour, some time, I will try to get a
better perspective on my life.

Just for Today I will be unafraid. Especially
I will not be afraid to enjoy what is beautiful,
and to believe as I give to the world, so the
world will give to me.

Start Your Day the Greysheet Way

1. We admitted we were powerless over food and that our lives had become unmanageable

2. Came to believe that a Power greater than ourselves could restore us to sanity

3. Made a decision to turn our will and out lives over to the care of God as we understood Him

11.Sought through Prayer and meditation to improve our conscious contact with God as we understood Him, praying only for knowledge of His will for us and the power to carry that out.

The Serenity Prayer
God grant me the serenity to accept
The things I cannot change; the courage to
Change the things I can, and the wisdom
To know the difference.

If We Don't Take That First Bite Today...
We'll never take it, because it's always today.

Look To This Very Day For It Is Life

There Are Two Days In Every Week
About which we should not worry
two days which should be kept from
fear and apprehension.
One of these days is yesterday. With
its mistakes and cares, its faults
and blunders, its aches and pains.
Yesterday has passed forever, beyond
our control. All the money in the
World cannot undo a single act we
performed. We cannot erase a single
word we said.

Yesterday is gone.

The other day we should not worry about is tomorrow.
With its possible adversaries, its burdens, its large promise and poor performance. Tomorrow is also beyond our immediate control.
Tomorrow's sun will rise either in splender or behind a mask of clouds-
But it will rise.

Until it does, we have not stake in tomorrow, for it is as yet unborn.

This leave only one day–Today.
any man can fight the battle of Just one day. It is only when you and I add the burden of those two awful eternities–yesterday and tomorrow that we break down.

It is not the experience of today that drives men mad, it is the remorse of bitterness, something which happened yesterday, and the dread of what tomorrow may bring.

Let us therefore live but
One Day At a Time!
And leave the rest to God

Love Is Friendship
that Has Caught Fire.
It is quiet understanding, mutual confidence, sharing and forgiving. It is loyalty through good times and bad. It settles for less than perfection and makes allowances for human weaknesses.

Love is content with the present; it hopes for the future, and it doesn't brood over the past. It's the day-in-day-out chronicles of irritations, problems, compromises, small disappointments, big victories and common goals.

If you have love in your life, it can make up for a great many things you lack. If you don't have it, no matter what else there is, it's not enough.

Before you Eat, Pick Up the Phone

This Is Home
And You Are Too Old
To Run Away from Home

Resources

GreySheeters Anonymous World Services (GSA) official website:
http://www.greysheet.org/

Literature

AA Conference-Approved Literature

Big Book, Alcoholics Anonymous, AA World Services, Inc.
Online, 4th Edition; Anonymous Press
International Journal of AA: AA Grapevine - AA's Meeting In Print "Box 1980"
12 & 12, Twelve Steps and Twelve Traditions
Living Sober (#2150)
A.A. Comes of Age (B-3)
As Bill Sees It (B-5)
Came To Believe (B-6)
Dr. Bob and the Good Oldtimers (B-8)
Pass It On (B-9)
Daily Reflections (B-12)
The Language of the Heart. Available for purchase at your local AA Meeting, Central Office, or Intergroup

Other Recovery Literature

From Hazelden *http://www.hazelden.org*

Little Red Book
Stools And Bottles
Twenty Four Hours A Day

Online Groups & Greysheet-Related Websites

GreyNet - An online forum for discussing the basics of attaining and maintaining GreySheet abstinence from compulsive eating.
http://health.groups.yahoo.com/group/greynet/
GreyNet Men's Meeting - An online forum where Men can discuss the basics of attaining and maintaining GreySheet abstinence from compulsive eating by following the GreySheet food plan, taking the 12 Steps, and sharing our experience, strength, and hope.
http://health.groups.yahoo.com/group/Greynet_The_Mens_Meeting/
Don't Eat No Matter What - An interactive online book; a community solution for compulsive overeating. *http://www.donteatnomatterwhat.com/*
GSA Phone Bridge Meetings Intergroup - A partnership of individual GSA Phone Bridge Meetings established to carry out certain functions common to all phone bridge meetings.
http://health.groups.yahoo.com/group/GSA_PBM_IG/
GreySheet Recipes Yahoo! Group - An online forum for members to post and discuss recipes that meet the requirements of the GreySheet food plan.
http://groups.yahoo.com/group/GreysheetRecipes/
GreysheetRecipes Website - Greysheet Recipes for free Download of Greysheet Rrecipes Collection and information for ordering printed copies of the Greysheet Recipes Collection. *http://www.greysheetrecipes.org*.

• GSA Northwest - Puget Sound, Seattle areas of Washington, and Oregon
http://www.greysheetnw.org/

• GSA San Diego - San Diego, California
http://www.greysheetsandiego.org

• Paris, France - 12 Step Meetings, including GreySheet
http://www.chez.com/groupesdeparis/

GSA Phone Meetings

Schedule *http://www.greysheet.org/meetphon.shtml*
Format *http://www.greysheet.org/gsphonemeetform.shtml*

Scales

Old Will Knott's Scales - *http://www.oldwillknott.com/*
MyScale.com - ScaleWorks, Gram Precision, Ohaus brands; call 866-222-2291. *http://www.myscale.com/*
Measurement Specialties, Inc. - Portion Power and Thinner brands. *http://www.clorders.com/measurementspecfoodscale.htm*
Tanita 1475 - weighs in ounces or grams. *http://www.scaleman.com/tanita/*
Nutritional Designs Labs, Inc. - Soehnle scales; or call Beth at 888-2ND-LABS; or email *sales@ndlabs.com. http://ndlabs.com/*
American Weigh - American Weigh, Escali, Ohaus, Salter, Tanita, My Weigh brands. *http://www.americanweigh.com/*

Soy Products - Check all ingredients with your sponsor/

ND Labs, Inc. - TVP, 4 flavors of soy nuts, wheat germ; call Beth at 1-888-2ND-LABS; or email *sales@ndlabs.com. http://ndlabs.com/*
Healthy Eating - TVP, soy nuts, tofu, soy beans, soy milk, soy nut butter *http://www.healthy-eating.com/*
Something Better Natural Foods - roasted/unroasted, salted/unsalted soy nuts, onion/garlic flavored; or call 616-965-1199; FAX 616-965-8500. *http://www.somethingbetternaturalfoods.com/*
SoSoya+ - dehydrated soy products in slices and ground; unsalted and sea salted organic dry roasted soy nuts; or call 416-293-6555; FAX 416-293-6459; or email *info@portello.com. http://www.so-soya.com/*
NOW Foods - textured soy protein (tsp), soybeans, instant soy milk powder, soy grits, certified organic, raw soy flour, soy powder, dry roasted, unsalted & salted soybeans, also onion & garlic, cajun, & BBQ flavored soynuts; or call 800-EAT-TOFU or 800-999-8069. *http://www.nowfoods.com/*
Soy Noodles - Sun Hing Food Co., 5505 N. Broadway, Chicago, IL, 773-728-6556, FAX 773-728-7453.

Soy Product descriptions:

Abstinent and Vegan

Soy Beans - black and white; hot or cold; dried that need soaking and cooking, or already cooked in cans. Westbrae (*http://www.westbrae.com/products/org_beans/osyb.html*) makes canned, organic soybeans. Just open and rinse the gel off with hot water. Eden Foods (*http://www.edenfoods.com/HostedStore.LassoApp?-ResponseLassoApp=search.lasso&ProductName=Black%20Soybeans,%20Organic*) makes canned, black organic soybeans.

Fresh Green Soybeans ("Edamame") - similar to green peas; available in pods or already shelled; usually frozen, but sometimes available fresh in Asian stores. Seapoint Farms, (*http://www.seapointfarms.com/products.asp?cat=42&hierarchy=0*) Sunrich, (*http://www.sunrich.com/hn/products/edamame/*) Melissa's World Variety Produce, (*http://www.melissas.com/catalog/index.cfm?Product_id=634&Info=YES*) Northland Organic (http://www.northlandorganic.com/organic/english/edamame.html)

Soy Milk - soaked, cooked soybeans that are ground, pressed, and filtered into a milk. Unopened, aseptically packaged soymilk can be stored at room temperature for several months. Once it is opened, the soymilk must be refrigerated. It will stay fresh for about 5 days. Soymilk is also sold as a powder, which must be mixed with water. Soymilk powder should be stored in the refrigerator or freezer. You can buy the powder and make your own so that you are sure there is no sweetener added. Eden Foods (*http://www.edenfoods.com/HostedStore.LassoApp?-ResponseLassoApp=search.lasso&ProductName=Black%20Soybeans,%20Organic* and WestSoy (*http://www.westsoy.biz/products/organic.php*) make unsweetened, plain varieties. Beware of "plain" varieties that still contain rice syrup, cane juice, and other sweeteners.

Soy Cheese - vegan without casein (a protein from the lining of calves stomachs in most "vegetarian" soy cheeses).

Tofu - firm, medium, soft; fresh or cooked; blended into "yogurt", dip, or spread; fried, marinated, flavored, etc.

Baked Tofu sold at Whole Foods, etc. Several flavors such as BBQ, Thai, etc.

Fried Tofu is available in thick squares or triangles or thin strips and there are many brands.

Tofu "Egg Salads" and other great imitation salads sold by Whole Foods, etc.

Soybean "Pasta" comes in strips or sheets so you can make imitation spaghetti or lasagna, or wrap vegetables like egg rolls. Read labels carefully. New soy pastas are being marketed that have semolina or flour high on the list of ingredients. Nutrition Kitchen (http://www.nutrikitchen.com/soybean_pasta.html) makes soy pasta that is 100% Certified Organic Whole Soybeans.

Miso - aged and fermented soybean paste - sort of like solid soy sauce - great for flavoring TVP or tofu. Like tempeh, it is often mixed with grains, so be careful to get "hacho" miso - just the soybeans.

Thit Chay - pure soybeans - no other ingredient. It looks like pork rinds or cheese doodles and comes dark or light in 4 oz. bags that look like single serving potato chip bags. They are meant to be soaked in water and then used as a meat substitute in recipes.

Tempeh - soy tempeh rather than vegetable, rice, or other grain tempeh - again, may be eaten fresh out of the pack, or cooked in many ways, such as crumbled or stir fried in slices. Really good microwaved until crunchy.

TVP, SVP, Soy Chunks, or Soy Nuggets, etc - defatted and either flaked, crumbled, or chunked soybeans. It comes flavored (lots of imitation meat flavors, like chicken, beef, turkey, etc) or plain. It can be eaten dry or soaked in water, sweetened or flavored. Some eat it dry with soymilk like a breakfast cereal. TSP, textured soy protein, is produced from soy flour after the soybean oil has been extracted, then cooked under pressure, extruded, and dried.

Soy Flour, Fermented Soy Flour, Soy Powder, and Soy Granules (although not sponsored by some sponsors) can be used to bake all kinds of imaginative things.

Meat Analogs made with soy - hot dogs, frankfurters, sausages, bacon, hamburgers, chorizo, taco mix, etc. Watch out for casein and sugar, grain, or vegetable ingredients.

Soy Nuts. Halved, dry roasted (light) or whole, roasted in fat (dark). These also come flavored (Salsa, BBQ, Cheese, Onion, etc) and either salted or not. These are becoming extremely common and appear in grocery stores and drug stores now.

Soy Margarine

Soy Puffs sold by Super Stop and Shop stores, made by Azumaya. The ingredients are water, soybeans, soy oil and baking soda. They come in a package of three. Zap them for three minutes in microwave and add soy butter.

Soy Nut Butter - comes in low carb, unsweetened crunchy or low carb, unsweetened creamy varieties. Read labels carefully.. I.M. Healthy Soy Nut Butter (*http://www.soynutbutter.com/product.html*)

Soy Bran - so far only found in the UK and delivered to the US by kind English GSers. Only ingredient is soy. Adds a nutty flavor to items baked with soy flour.

Soy Chips - come in chicken and other flavors and various sizes and shapes. Can be eaten crunchy and dry or soaked in liquid and cooked like meat.

Soy Chicken - fantastic flavor and consistency. Comes in refrigerated section of Asian grocery stores in 12-ounce packages as one piece (looking like a chicken breast) or chicken nuggets.

SoSoya+ - Dried soy product that comes in stir-fry sized "slices," at Trader Joe's. It's expensive, but it makes a fabulous stay-crunchy cereal.

Abstinent and Vegetarian But Not Vegan:

Tofu Pudding - from Plum Flower available in Asian grocery stores. It is apparently just like custard in consistency without any taste at all. You can add fruit or other tastes. It has gelatin so it isn't vegan.

Soy Cheese - varieties that contain casein include: Yves Veggie. (*http://www.yvesveggie.com/splash.php?referer=products_family.php&refererQS=family_id%3D8%26page%3D1%26pId%3DlItem9%26pIdName%3DGood%2520Slices*)

Soy Cream Cheese, Soy Cottage Cheese, Soy Sour Cream, and Soy Yogurt - all seem to have casein.

Soy Cookies - from Soybite. Abstinent flavors include plain, coffee, peanut butter (8th ingredient), and chocolate chip. Available in NYC at Natural Frontier. Six packages for $19.99 online.

Original Flavored Soy "Tortilla" Chips - by Keto (ranch and nacho cheese flavors). Available at GNC and Natural Frontier in New York City. Vitacost (*http://www.vitacost.com/*) and Spinelli's (*http://www.spinellinutrition.com/keto-tortilla-chips.html*) sell these.

Extracts - Flavorings - Coffees - Alcohol-Free, Sugar-Free - Check extract use with your sponsor.

Bickford Flavors - or call 800-283-8322 and request a brochure.
http://www.bickfordflavors.com/
Da Vinci's - Splenda-Sweetened Flavored Syrups
http://www.davincigourmet.com/729.html?flashdetect=YES
Dolce - Nutra-Sweetened Flavored Syrups *http://www.coffeeam.com/*
Frontier Co-op - listed as "Natural Flavors"; or call 800-786-1388 and request a catalog.
http://www.frontiercoop.com/shop/merchant.mvc?Store_Code=FNPC
Frontier Co-op - culinary spices, seasoning blends
http://www.frontiercoop.com/shop/merchant.mvc?Store_Code=FNPC
Nature's Flavors - bulk herbs and spices *http://www.naturesflavors.com/*
Nature's Flavors -listed as "Flavor Concentrates".
http://www.naturesflavors.com/
ND Labs, Inc. - listed as "Extracts"; or call Beth at 1-888-2ND-LABS; or *email sales@ndlabs.com. http://ndlabs.com/*
Penzeys Spices - spices, herbs, and seasonings; gift boxes, specialty spices; mills and containers *http://www.naturesflavors.com/*

Spices Etc. - herbs, spices, and seasonings; storage and usage tips; grinders, racks, gifts
http://www.spicesetc.com/

Coffee Syrups - Alcohol-Free, Sugar-Free - Check syrup use with your sponsor.

Barnie's Coffee & Tea Company - light, medium, dark roasted; flavored, decaf; black and green teas *http://www.barniescoffee.com/ecomm/Home.jsp*
coffeeAM - original, organic, and decaf flavored coffees; gourmet teas; coffee of the month club *http://www.coffeeam.com/*
Coffee Specialties - premium flavored gourmet coffees, city roast, select varietals, euromild acid reduced, Hawaiian, Jamaican, organic *http://www.coffeespecialties.com/*
Coffees and Teas *http://www.coffeewholesalers.com/*
Cook's Corner - gourmet coffee, flavored coffee, varieties, blends, and dark roasts *http://www.cookscorner.net/*
Nature's Flavors - Splenda-Sweetened Flavored Syrups *http://www.naturesflavors.com/*
Torani - Splenda-Sweetened Flavored Syrups

Spices - Check spice use with your sponsor.

Restaurants - Greysheet Friendly to Measuring

"Grace's" Chinese restaurant in NYC - Sung Chu Mei, 212-675-0016, 615 Hudson St. near 12th & Jane in Greenwich Village

Sugar & Sweetner Labeling

Names for Sugar and Other Sweeteners
This is a partial list of various names for sugar or other sweeteners compiled as a service for GreySheeters who want to avoid these substances. Not all of these items are non-abstinent, i.e., some of the items may be abstinent for some people, for example Stevia. Check with your sponsor.

Barbados Sugar
Barley Malt
Beet Juice
Beet Sugar
Black Strap Molasses
Brown Rice Syrup (In Most Soy Milks)
Brown Sugar
Cane Sugar
Cane Syrup

Caramel
Carob Powder
Confectioner's Sugar
Cooked Honey
Corn Starch
Corn Sugar
Corn Sweetener
Corn Syrup
Crystalline Carbohydrate
Crystalline Fructose
Dark Brown Sugar
Date Sugar
Date Syrup
Demerara (British)
Dextrin
Dextrose
Disaccharides
Evaporated/Crystallized Cane Juice
Fig Syrup
Filtered Honey
Fructose
Fruit Juice Concentrate (All Types)
Fruit Nectars
Fruit Sugar
Fruit Sweetener
Galactose
Glucose
Glyco-
Golden Brown Sugar
Granulated Sugar
Grape Sugar
Grape Sweetener
Heavy Syrup
HFCS
High Fructose Corn Syrup
Honey
Hydrogenated Glucose Syrup
Invert Sugar
Jaggery
Juice Concentrate
Lactose
Lactose (Milk Sugar)
Levulose (Fruit Sugar)
Light Brown Sugar
Light Sugar
Light Syrup
Lite Syrup
Lo-Sugar
Low Sugar
Malt
Malt Syrup
Malted
Malted Barley
Malted Syrup
Maltitol
Malto-(Anything Else)
Maltodextrin
Maltose (Malt Sugar)
Manitol
Mannitol
Maple Sugar
Maple Syrup
Molasses
Mono-Saccharides
Muscavado (Barbados Sugar)
Natural Sweeteners
Natural Syrup
Polydextrose
Polysaccharides
Poly-Saccharides
Powdered Sugar
Raisin Syrup
Raw Honey
Raw Sugar
Raw Sugar or Turbinado Sugar
Ribbon Cane Syrup
Ribose
Rice Malts
Rice Syrup
Rum

Sorbitol
Sorghum
Sorghum Molasses
Sorghum Syrup
Starch Syrup
Stevia
Suamiel
Succanat
Sucrose (Table Sugar)
Sugar
Sugar Alcohols (Ex. Mannitol, Sorbitol, Xylitol)
Sugar Cane Syrup
Syrups (Ex. Maple, Sorghum)
Table Sugar
Turbinado
Uncooked Honey
White Sugar
Xylitol

This resource list is not an official GSA publication. Information has been supplied by individual GreySheeters for informational purposes only. The appearance of resources and hyperlinks on this page does not constitute endorsement by Greysheet Recipes or GreySheeters Anonymous World Services, Inc. of web sites or the information, products, or services contained therein.

Index

COOKED VEGETABLE WITH PROTEIN 141

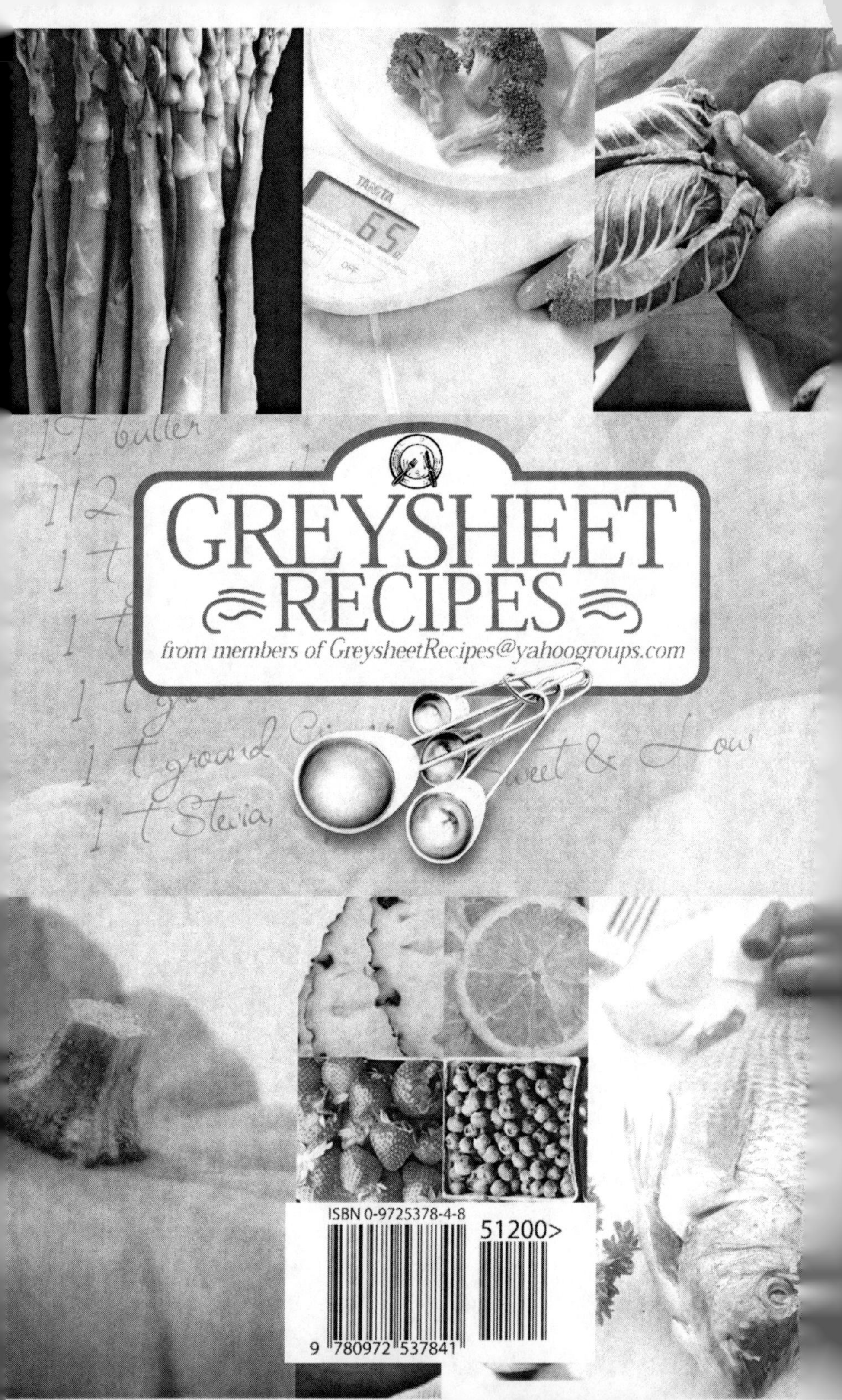

GREYSHEET
RECIPES
from members of GreysheetRecipes@yahoogroups.com
1 T butter
1/2
1 t
1 t
1 t
1 t ground
1 t Stevia,
Sweet & Low
ISBN 0-9725378-4-8
51200>
9 780972 537841

CPSIA information can be obtained at www.ICGtesting.com
Printed in the USA
LVOW051520180812

294901LV00001B/268/P